Agua Albino poo Alfie Amp Annie Barn͏ͅ Batu kilat Batu Batunas Beans Bennies Bonz Blanca Biker dope Billy Bitch Blanco Blizzard Blue acid Blue funk Bomb Booger or booger sugar Boorit cebuano Boo-ya Bug Bumps Buzzard dust C.C.C.R. Ca-ca Candy Cha cha cha Chach Chalk or chalk dust Chameleon Chank Cheebah Cheese Chicken Chingadera Chittle Chizel Chiznad Choad Chrissy or Christy Clavo Coco Coffee Cookies Crank Crankenstein Cri-cri Criddle Cringe Critty Crotch dope Crow Crunk Crypto Crystal Crystal light Crystal meth Cube or ice cube Debbie Devil dust Devil's dandruff Devil's drug Dex Diet pills Dingle Dirt or dirty Dizzy-DD-monic Doo-dah Doody Dope Drano Dummy dust Dyno Epod Eraser dust Ethyl-M Fatch Fedrin Fizz wizz Flash, Gack Gas Gemini Glass Go Go-fast Go-go or go-go juice Gonzalez Goop Grit Gumption Gyp Hank Hawaiian Salt High-speed chicken feed Hillbilly crack or hippie crack Homework Hoo Horse mumpy Hydro Ice Ice cream Ish Izice Jab Jasmine Jenny crank program Jet fuel Jib Jinga Juddha Juice Junk Kibble Killer Kool-aid Kryptonite L.A. Lamer Laundry detergent Lemon drop Life Lily Linda Love Low Lucille Magic Meth Methane Methanfelony Methatrim Methlé's quick Method Mexican crack Motivation Nazi dope Ned New Prozac No Doze Nose candy Patsie Peanut butter Pepsi Phazers Phets Philopon Pieta Pink Poison Poop Poor man's cocaine Powder PowderPoint Propellant Puddle Pump Quartz Quick Quill Rails Rank Redneck heroin Richie Rich Rip Rock Rocket fuel Rocky Mountain high Rosebud Sack Satan dust Scap Scooby snacks Scud Shabu Shards She-bang Shit Shiznit Shizzo Shwack Skeech Sketch Ski Skitz Sky rocks Sliggers Smiley Snaps Sniff Snow Space food Spaceman Sparkle Speed Speed Racer Spin Spinderella Spinny boo Spokane Spook Sprack Sprung Squawk Stovetop Sugar Sweetness Swerve Tacoma Talkie Tasmanian Devil Tenner Tina Tish Toots Trash Tubbytoast Tutu Tweak Wake-up Walk White White bitch White crunch White house White junk White lady White pony Whizz Ya ba Zoom

ICED

CRYSTAL METH: THE BIOGRAPHY OF
NORTH AMERICA'S DEADLIEST NEW PLAGUE

JERRY LANGTON

KEY PORTER BOOKS

Library and Archives Canada Cataloguing in Publication

Langton, Jerry, 1965–
· Iced: crystal meth: the biography of north america's deadliest new plague / Jerry Langton.

ISBN-13: 978-1-55263-831-6
ISBN-10: 1-55263-831-6

1. Ice (Drug). 2. Methamphetamine abuse. I. Title.

HV5822.A5L35 2007   362.29'9   C2006-901815-4

The publisher gratefully acknowledges the support of the Canada Council for the Arts and the Ontario Arts Council for its publishing program. We acknowledge the support of the Government of Ontario through the Ontario Media Development Corporation's Ontario Book Initiative.

We acknowledge the financial support of the Government of Canada through the Book Publishing Industry Development Program (BPIDP) for our publishing activities.

Distributed in the U.S. by Publishers Group West
www.pgw.com

Key Porter Books Limited
Six Adelaide Street East, Tenth Floor
Toronto, Ontario
Canada M5C 1H6

www.keyporter.com

Text design: Marijke Friesen
Electronic formatting: Jean Lightfoot Peters

Printed and bound in Canada

07 08 09 10 11 5 4 3 2 1

TABLE OF CONTENTS

To Tonia and
the Greasy Thugs

INTRODUCTION

E VERY SOCIETY has a hierarchy.

I was sharply reminded of that fact when I was leaving a seedy bar in Hamilton, Ontario, and the people I was interviewing started making fun of a guy on the street. Eddie was just hanging around outside the bar—not bothering anybody—but he did have a weak, vulnerable look about him. As soon as my associates saw him, they started in on him. It began quietly at first, but when it began to become more fun, it got worse. Most of their insults were about how low he'd sunk, about how many "dicks he'd sucked" that night. Eddie took it all good-naturedly and pathetically tried to keep an amiable look on his face.

Keep in mind that the guys I was with—the tormentors—all either smoked or sold crack cocaine (most, I suspected, did both). The reason they all felt superior to Eddie was that they all felt they could control their drug use and they knew very well he couldn't. The difference was that Eddie was addicted to meth. And meth addicts are at the bottom of the drug-using heap.

While I was writing my first book—*Fallen Angel: The Unlikely Rise of Walter Stadnick and the Canadian Hells Angels*—I learned a few truisms of the drug trade. One is that nobody, but nobody, is considered sadder and more lost than a hardcore meth addict. Another is that meth is remarkably easy to sell. One dealer even told me that he could "sell meth wherever there are white people."

That's just one of the strange and dangerous ironies of meth. A shocking number of people, perhaps confusing meth with the chemically similar stimulants from a generation or two ago, will give it a try. It's usually a lot cheaper than cocaine and easier to get. And the sales pitch is hard to beat—meth really does make you happy, thin, ambitious and sexy.

But perhaps less well-known is the fact that meth use is often followed by a hangover that could make the most jaded alcoholic contemplate suicide. After prolonged use, there's no way to make the pain go away—except for more meth and, after that stops working, the pain, the feelings of worthlessness, self-loathing and paranoia may never actually go away.

That's why I wanted to write *Iced*. My research for *Fallen Angel* and other stories showed me how utterly disastrous meth can be to lives, families and even whole communities. As I wrote it, though, I came across a surprising number of opinions in the mainstream media that suggested meth was not an epidemic; that other publications—most notably *Newsweek*—were fear-mongering and pushing the idea to boost sales. I have to disagree, and I think that's why *Iced* is necessary.

While it's absolutely true that any drug can ruin lives, my observations have convinced me that meth does it more effectively than any of the others. I've yet to come across a serious commentator who disagrees with that, of course. Instead, they deny that meth is so widespread and as prevalent as to be considered an epidemic. That's because you have to go looking for it. You won't find meth at the parties and nightclubs where cocaine sells. You won't see it written about in newspapers, because people don't overdose on it; they just fade away. And you won't find it in the largely black inner-city neighborhoods once ravaged by crack, where reporters occasionally go to prove their mettle.

Meth isn't like that. It's harder to pin down. The users aren't as easily identifiable. It might be the guy who changes your oil, it might be the woman who pours your coffee or it might be the kid who mows your lawn. It could be your pastor. And the people who take it never really want to talk about it—and some actually can't.

To get a better idea of what meth does and is doing, I spoke not just to users, but also to cops, health-care providers and the families of users. Yes, I know they all have agendas and axes to grind, but so does everybody. It's hard to find the truth about a subject as contentious as meth, but I think the only way to get close to it is to talk to the people who come into contact with it.

So instead of consulting drug-use surveys and talking to people in government, I went to the bars and corners where I knew people bought and sold drugs. I went to small towns, to flea markets and scrap yards. It wasn't glamorous; it wasn't easy and it sure wasn't fun.

When I went into the project, the one thing I didn't want it to be was like the way they show drug use on seventies-era cop shows. You know, the dealer seduces the user with wild promises, the user then gets hooked and becomes a pathetic slave to the drug. I may not have wanted it to be true, but often times it was.

I wrote *Iced* because I saw what meth could do to people. It's not a pretty picture.

WELCOME TO THE NEWEST PLAGUE

THE CRACKING IMPACT of the punch snapped her jaw sharply to the left.

Erin went straight down as though she'd slipped on ice. She couldn't see anything but a bright light, she recalled, and didn't know what had happened until she realized she was sitting on the floor staring up at Justin.

He was shaking, even hopping up and down a little bit, and looked wild. His face was pointed to the right, but his eyes, his wide, crazy eyes, were fixed straight at her. There was no guilt or remorse in his eyes, no hint of conscience. As much as she didn't want to believe it, she knew she'd been punched in the face and knocked to the floor by her only son. But what was far worse was the fact that she could tell from looking at him that if she got up, he'd probably do it again.

It's not like he was a bad kid. In fact, Justin had been a fairly quiet and reserved youngster who got average marks in school and rarely, if ever, got into trouble. That is, until he started taking meth. Erin had turned something of a blind eye to the fact that he had begun drinking when he was fifteen, mainly because, as she said, "he started a lot later than most of the kids around here." He hadn't gotten into any trouble and, although his grades suffered, Erin attributed that to his father leaving and other issues. She was sure he'd bounce back.

But he hadn't. Justin eventually dropped out of school and became a recluse. He'd lock himself in his bedroom for days at a time, doing God knows what, Erin remembers wondering, not

The North Dakota Department of Health has put together a convenient list of potential hazards for children born to mothers who use meth:

- Methamphetamine use during pregnancy affects development of a baby's brain, spinal cord, heart and kidneys.
- Methamphetamine use during pregnancy may result in prenatal complications, such as premature delivery and birth deformities.
- High doses of the drug may cause a baby's blood pressure to rise rapidly, leading them to suffer strokes or brain hemorrhages before birth.
- Babies whose mothers used methamphetamine during pregnancy may experience learning disabilities, growth and developmental delays.
- Methamphetamine-exposed babies may experience gastroschisis and other problems with the development of their intestines. (Gastroschisis is a condition in which a baby is born with a hole in the abdomen, causing the intestines to be outside the body.)
- As a result of methamphetamine use by their mothers, some babies may suffer developmental and skeletal abnormalities (such as clubfoot). Some babies are born without parts of their arms or legs.
- Because methamphetamine affects transmitters in the brain, babies often experience sleep disturbances and altered behavioral patterns. These babies have been described as "irritable babies."
- Full-term babies born to mothers who use methamphetamine will likely have difficulty sucking and swallowing, much like premature babies.
- Often babies born to meth-addicted women cannot tolerate stimuli such as human touch and light. These babies often display tremors and coordination problems.

eating, not communicating with the outside world at all. It got worse when he started leaving the house, sometimes for days on end. He'd come home, exhausted and sick-looking, and just sleep for hours and hours. He never said anything about where he went or what he was doing.

"I knew what was going on when he started taking my stuff and selling it," Erin said. "I knew it had to be an addictive drug—and from what happened to his body, it was pretty clear he was on speed."

Erin had gotten a call at work from a friend who recognized her TV at a nearby flea market. It was easy to spot because of a long crack in the plastic housing. Erin didn't know that it was missing, but wasn't actually all that surprised. After work, she went down to the market and explained what happened to the guy who was selling it.

"He said he understood and that he felt real bad," she said. "But he still made it clear that he didn't want to lose money on the deal. I guess I could have called the cops, but I gave him forty dollars—it was all I had on me."

When Justin came home, Erin decided it was finally time to confront him. He denied taking the set, but couldn't explain how it wound up at the flea market. At first, he tried to improvise a viable story. Then he just started babbling, which quickly escalated to shouting and then screaming.

That's when he smacked his mother in the face with a closed fist. Erin just sat there, she said, looking up at him blankly. Dumbfounded at first and then scared, she watched as he stalked off to his room and slammed the door behind him.

Erin was crying when she went to quit her job a few days later. A retail sales clerk at a housewares and home decorating store in a run-down little strip mall in an unimportant little southwestern Ontario town, the job had, nevertheless, meant a lot to her. It was a motivation to get up in the morning, a chance to meet people, a reason to feel good about herself. She'd been on welfare after her husband left her and wasn't happy about going down that road again. Erin didn't want to quit, but she knew she had to.

Her boss saved her the agony of having to go through with it. She told Erin that her job would be waiting for her whenever she was ready to come back. It's not like she was surprised, her boss had said. Everyone who knew Erin was aware of what was going on: Justin was back on the stuff. That he'd been getting into trouble again, fights mostly, but that he had also been shoplifting and stealing from his mother.

It wasn't until Justin punched his mother in the jaw that Erin knew she had to protect him. She didn't want to get the police involved because Justin had been in trouble with them before. "If he was arrested for this, judges would look at him like he was some kind of criminal and throw him in jail," she said. "And what good would jail do? Those places are crawling with drugs and he'd only make more bad friends there."

"It wasn't him anyway, it was the drugs," she said. "He was such a good boy until he got hooked on the crystal meth. Then he started to act like a monster."

Over the last few months Justin had started losing weight. He was staying up for three- and four-day stretches at a time. His mood was increasingly irritable and violent. He had developed painful lesions all over his face. He lost his job, his car, his girlfriend, his friends and most of his possessions.

Erin won't let him drive her old Nissan Sentra and hides her keys when she's asleep. "I'm afraid to let him drive," she told me. "It's not the accidents I'm afraid of. He's a good driver. I just think he'd go ahead and sell the damn thing."

Erin doesn't know what to do. Justin spends most of his time in bed or in the shower and when he gets up, he walks around like a zombie. He doesn't enjoy anything, cries often and has even lost the ability to read. She's looking after him, but she doesn't really know if she's actually helping him.

"It's like he's ninety years old," she said. "He depends on me for everything." Her options are limited. "I can't afford to pay for rehab, so I have him on the waiting list for a spot at the ministry," she shrugs, referring to government-subsidized rehab. She admits she doesn't have a great deal of faith in it.

"It's a long shot. I really don't know if he'll ever get better."

IN 2005 NEWSWEEK reported that 1.5 million Americans were regular meth users. A rhetorical—some would come to ask hysterical—headline screamed, "America's Most Dangerous Drug." Many sources report that more than 90 percent of those who try meth find themselves addicted to it a year later. The fact is, Justin is no different than hundreds of thousands of North Americans who have become hooked on crystal meth, a drug so powerful and so addictive it is widely blamed for the destruction of the social fabric of many large areas across the continent, particularly in the West.

Speed—as amphetamine-based stimulants are often called—has been around for decades and was, for much of the twentieth century, a stimulant commonly used to treat asthma, bronchitis, lethargy, narcolepsy, depression, hyperactivity and a variety of other ailments. It was such a common, and seemingly harmless, part of our lives that it was even sold as a diet supplement, allowing people to get more done and lose weight at the same time. Soldiers have been taking massive and regular doses of the stuff since the 1930s and many still do today, sanctioned by many governments including that of the U.S.

But doctors and police knew by the late 1940s that it was dangerous stuff and that users could turn psychotic if they took enough of it. Speed users didn't suffer the spectacular and headline-worthy overdoses heroin addicts did and they didn't try to fly out windows like LSD users were said to, so few media outlets, enforcement officials or politicians paid any significant attention to it. Instead, speed freaks (as they became known) simply wore down. They stopped eating and stopped sleeping. They died from depression- or psychosis-related suicides, or from hepatitis or even malnutrition.

But all of those drugs were later eclipsed by cocaine. First the darling of the jet set, cocaine became the "in" drug for achievers everywhere. It was, however, spectacularly expensive. Enterprising coke dealers wanted a larger market. They needed a cut-rate version of the drug. Named "crack" because of the cracking sound it made when lit, a new crystalline form of cocaine proved hugely popular. Retailing for as little as $5 a hit, crack made cocaine available to everyone. Happily for dealers and suppliers, crack was far more addictive than cocaine. Suddenly, hundreds of thousands of addicts desperate for more would find themselves doing whatever it took. All across North America crime rates skyrocketed. It was so bad that many American cities experienced a massive demographic shift as high- and middle-income people fled to the suburbs to escape the rampaging epidemic of crime perpetrated by desperate addicts, known as crackheads. After about a decade, crime rates fell precipitously—especially in large cities like New York—and people with money slowly began to return to the cities. There are a number of opinions as to why this happened. Some say that smarter, more efficient policing resulted in an environment hostile to petty crime. Others suggest that hardcore crackheads either died or went to prison and that the next generation of would-be users were so scared off of crack by what they'd seen that they never tried it.

Curiously, it's about that time that meth began showing up in volume.

Made from ephedrine, a chemical used in diet pills, or pseudoephedrine, the key ingredient in cold pills, meth was cheap
and plentiful to the point of being almost unlimited in supply.
Originally manufactured on farms and in remote areas by cooks
who jealously guarded their recipes, the stuff would later be
made by anyone who could find the instructions on the Internet
and who could buy some cold pills and lye.

Meth is a powder that resembles salt or a crack-like solid
(ice) that is odorless, bitter tasting, translucent and usually white
or yellowish. Occasionally, meth made in smaller labs will be red
or pink if the cook hasn't done a good job removing the dyed
coating from the cold pills. Rarely, meth will be available in pill
or capsule form, but few cooks, even in large operations called
superlabs, go to the trouble.

Traditional meth can be ingested in a variety of ways. It can
be swallowed, but the taste is pretty awful. Powdered meth is
often put into emptied-out capsules of over-the-counter cold
remedies or mixed into a beverage, most often orange juice or
coffee. Since it takes about twenty minutes for a user to feel the
affects of orally ingested meth, many turn to more immediate
methods.

It can be snorted like traditional cocaine, which cuts the wait
time to about five minutes. Some snort it straight from a table,
mirror or piece of glass, but most use straws, rolled-up paper
money or purpose-built devices. The crystals must be ground
(usually with a knife on a hard surface) into a fine powder, not
only because bigger chunks can irritate the nasal membranes,
but because they are harder to absorb and can go to waste. The
major problem with snorting meth is that it can quickly lead to
nasal congestion. Not only is that mildly unpleasant in and of
itself, it also inhibits the absorption of more meth. Prolonged
use can result in nasal irritation and even, if the meth is impure
enough, ulcers and perforations in the septum.

Somewhat more common is the practice of smoking meth like crack. Although I'm told the quickest highs (starting in as little as two or three minutes) come from inhaling the fumes of meth burned on foil (freebasing), on heated knife blades or on bent soda cans, most users consider these methods wasteful as much of the smoke is never inhaled. Although often little more than three to five inches of glass tubing, pipes can be quite elaborate, often using water chambers to help filter out impurities. Of course, smoking meth carries the same dangers that come along with smoking any drug. The user could be inhaling the smoke of any of a number of different poisonous, corrosive and potentially carcinogenic substances.

Knowledgeable users have told me that since meth disappears very quickly when it's smoked and the high is so intense, people who smoke the drug tend to buy more and get hooked more quickly. There's no scientific documentation to back that hypothesis up, but it seems to be a widely held opinion.

Traditionally much less popular, intravenous use of meth is rapidly growing and, in some parts of North America, now accounts for the majority of use. For intravenous use, meth is dissolved and injected directly into a blood vessel with a syringe. The high is almost immediate and the most intense of all methods.

Air bubbles in the injection, however, can cause intense pain and even death. Sharing needles is a remarkably efficient way to spread diseases like Hepatitis B and C, tuberculosis and HIV. The popularity of meth in the gay community has had a devastating impact.

"Effective treatment for methamphetamine-related drug disorders may be one of the most important strategies in reducing the spread of HIV and other associated communicable infections," says Richard A. Rawson, Ph.D., associate director, UCLA Integrated Substance Abuse Programs, UCLA School of Medicine, and one of the world's foremost experts on meth use. "Among heterosexual, injection methamphetamine users, Hepatitis C rates of approximately 50 to 60 percent have been reported."

Experts generally agree that intravenous meth users are likely to be the most addicted and the most desperate of all meth addicts. "Methamphetamine use (especially injection use) has also been highly associated with participation in illegal behaviors, such as crime and violence," says Rawson.

Ironically, as dangerous as meth was proving to be, it lacked the ugly social stigma associated with crack and crack addiction, and the drug found a willing population of users essentially unaware of its dangers. An addict I spoke with said that at first she had confused meth with amphetamines, which she thought were "sort of a harmless thing from back in the hippie days."

She was wrong. That innocuous prefix that separates methamphetamine from amphetamine is profoundly important. Scientifically, it means that it has a molecular compound that makes it bond more quickly to other chemicals. Prosaically, it means that it works faster and much more effectively. A man who considered himself something of a drug connoisseur and had used both told me the difference was a like "a pop gun compared to an atomic bomb." The first time you use meth, it gives an intense rush that simply can't be equaled by anything else. Your brain sends all of its feel-good chemicals out at once and the flood is absolutely overwhelming.

"Immediate physiological changes associated with methamphetamine use are similar to those produced by the fight-or-flight response, inducing increased blood pressure, body temperature, heart rate and breathing," says Rawson. "Even small doses can increase wakefulness, attention, and physical activity and decrease fatigue and appetite." It acts like adrenaline, the naturally occurring hormone that allows people to function under highly stressful conditions.

While that first super-intense high only lasts for a few minutes, meth keeps on supplying the body with a surge for eight to twelve hours, far longer than cocaine, which can be entirely metabolized in as little as twenty minutes. During this secondary, prolonged high, users feel marked increases in alertness, motivation, talkativeness, confidence and self-esteem.

It was this "surge" in hormones that led to its increased use by those in highly stressful situations, such as entertainers, harried students preparing for exams, even athletes. Moderate doses can ward off sleep for days, which made meth use popular with truck drivers, pilots and other people who needed to stay awake and alert for long, otherwise tedious stretches. And the increased energy and suppression of appetite appealed to many people who wanted to lose weight quickly.

The drug's greatest selling point, however, may be the fact that it greatly increases sexual stimulation and desire in both sexes. One former second-grade teacher told a Phoenix newspaper that her meth addiction made her quit her job, become a stripper and then later a prostitute—and not just because of the money. In a period of less than two years, she estimated that she had sex with well over two thousand men—"mostly unprotected"—and many women. Even though she was almost constantly selling sex for meth money, she still spent most of her spare time having sex with herself.

"I would masturbate for eight hours straight," she said. "I remember once that the dildo I was using got so hot, I had to wear an oven mitt."

The primary physical side effects of meth use, even from the first dose, include high blood pressure, rapid heartbeat, headaches, irregular heartbeat and nausea.

"The psychological impact is manifested by increased anxiety, insomnia, aggression and violent tendencies, paranoia and visual and auditory hallucinations," says Rawson. "High doses can elevate body temperature to dangerous, sometimes lethal levels, causing convulsions, coma, stroke and vegetative states and even death."

For most users, the rush and the buzz far outweigh any unpleasant side effects. Kyle, a frequent user I know, told me that if he suffered any side effects he didn't notice them because he was "too busy enjoying the high." It was so good, he told me, that before it had worn off he was already wondering when he could get his next hit.

"Prolonged use of methamphetamine frequently creates tolerance for the drug and escalating dosage levels creates dependence," says Rawson. "As tolerance occurs, users typically increase the methamphetamine dose and increase the frequency of use." That tolerance very quickly begins to dull the high but does nothing to quell the many symptoms of withdrawal, which often get even more intolerable. The only cure for a meth hangover is more meth.

Casual "recreational" users quickly become addicts. The majority of experts agree that meth is more addictive even than crack. The most commonly repeated statistics are that 98 percent of first-time meth users become addicted after a year, and that no more than 6 percent of addicts are ever able to kick the drug in any meaningful way.

The United Nations Office of Drug Control estimates that there are about 42 million users of meth and related drugs worldwide, more than any other illegal drug except marijuana and at least double that of those use cocaine and four times that of those who use heroin. The Substance Abuse and Mental Health Services Administration (SAMHSA), a branch of the U.S. Department of Health and Human Services, reports that admissions to its rehab centers for meth-related problems grew 420 percent between 1993 and 2005.

"In some states, methamphetamine has emerged as the most significant drug problem within the treatment system. Treatment

admission rates for persons aged twelve years and older have drastically risen over the past decade from 10 per 100,000 in 1992 to
52 per 100,000 in 2002," says Rawson. "In 2002, fourteen states
cited that there were more admissions resulting from methamphetamine use than from heroin and cocaine use combined, and
recent data reveal that methamphetamine admissions increased
10 percent between 2002 and 2003."

Repeated use of the drug usually results in violent behavior,
anxiety, confusion and insomnia.

"These symptoms are the combined result of direct drug
effects plus the consequences associated with sleep deprivation,
as abusers will often report days and even weeks of sleeplessness," says Rawson. "When in a state of prolonged
methamphetamine use and sleep deprivation, users commonly
experience a number of psychotic features, including paranoia,
auditory hallucinations, mood disturbances and delusions."

One of the most frequently reported side effects of long-
term meth use is delusional parasitosis—the belief that insects
or other vermin are crawling on or just under the user's skin.
Also known as "formication" (from the Latin word *formica*,
which means ant) or Ekborn's Syndrome (after the neurologist
who first published accounts of it in the 1930s), the concept has
been used as a comedic device by author Hunter S. Thompson
and *Doonesbury* cartoonist Garry Trudeau. But it can have serious consequences as those affected scratch, pick and even take
knives and other tools to their skin in an effort to get at their
imaginary tormentors.

"The bad ones always have sores and lesions from picking at
their skin," says a paramedic I spoke with. "They really think the
bugs are there and there's no way to convince them they aren't."

More commonplace and somewhat more frightening than
delusional parasitosis is *anhedonia*, the total lack of ability to
feel happiness. Because frequent meth users keep overloading

the receptors and pathways in their brains that accept the feel-good hormones, they can become damaged or even destroyed. The result is that the brain loses the capacity to signal pleasure no matter what the stimuli. Things that normally feel good and satisfying—food, sex, companionship—simply can't be appreciated anymore.

"Justin doesn't do anything anymore, just sits there and stares," Erin says of her son. "I knew it was bad when he stopped playing video games. I have to force him to eat because he tells me he can't taste anything anymore."

Some of the psychosis suffered by long-term meth users is externalized and erupts in violence and criminal behavior. When high they feel self-confident to the point of invincibility. When they are hungover, however, they are desperate for another hit. Sometimes, obsessively so.

Users generally experience a remarkable increase in libido. Statistics show that the primary population of meth users for sexual purposes have been gay men.

"When consumed in sexually-charged environments like dance parties, saunas and sex clubs, the focus on sex can become compulsive and create a sense of hypersexuality," reads a report on lifeormeth.com, a website dedicated to recovery targeted primarily at the gay community, "opening the user to previously unrealized and extreme desires. Crystal's compatibility with reckless, furious, hedonistic, no-strings-attached sex—combined with an increased duration of arousal and inability to ejaculate—paved the way for intensive sex marathons with multiple partners lasting up to several days."

Not only does meth increase the sex drive, it makes users a lot more casual about having sex. According to a 2001 study of HIV-positive men who use meth, 84 percent reported engaging in what many would consider risky sexual behavior. The majority of them declined to reveal their HIV status to their casual partners, the report states, and many reported that they assumed their sex partners to be HIV-positive unless they were informed otherwise upfront.

According to the U.S. Department of Health and Human Services, reported cases of gonorrhea and syphilis, often thought to be good indicators of future HIV levels, are steadily rising among gay men—especially among meth users.

"We've compared meth to cocaine, opiates and alcohol, and have found much more of a connection between sex and meth than those other drugs," said Rawson. "It increases sexual pleasure, it increases sexual activity, and it increases the extreme kinds of high-risk behavior that lead to HIV and other STDs. More so than any other drug."

Prolonged meth use, however, can have adverse effects on the sex drive. Users often experience a problem known universally as "crystal dick" in which they have a difficult time maintaining or even achieving an erection.

"It's most likely the result of vein damage and changes in brain chemicals that cause an erection," says a spokesman for Stonewall Recovery Services, a not-for-profit organization that promotes health issues for gay men. "Sometimes, these changes are permanent."

Many men combat crystal dick with the anti-impotence drug Viagra. There are differences of opinion as to whether it works or not, but there is no disagreement that both drugs have profound effects on both blood pressure and heart rate, and that taking them together can be fatal.

Because it is such an effective appetite suppressant, meth use does cause weight loss, often immediately. It also stimulates and increases energy and motivation. Long-term meth users, however, can develop a bizarre skeletal appearance. Accentuating that wasted look is the fact that prolonged use can lead to accelerated tooth decay—a syndrome widely known as "meth mouth." Because of various factors, including a lack of saliva, teeth clenching and grinding and a lack of blood supply to the gums, long-term meth users often have horrific smiles full of broken and missing teeth.

Even those people foolish enough to take their chances with the long-term destructive effects of the drug should realize that when they're ingesting meth, that's not all they're getting. Even the best meth from the Mexican superlabs is no better than 70 percent pure, and much of what is produced in smaller labs is reported to be closer to half that. At the retail level, meth is often cut with talcum powder, salt, sugar, Prozac, protease inhibitors, Ritalin, laxatives, Epsom salts or anything else handy that can pass for meth. These impurities are intentionally added in an effort to stretch out the supply—like putting breadcrumbs into a meatloaf.

Potentially worse is the toxic residue left behind by the manufacturing process. Most meth recipes include ingredients like battery acid, hydrochloric acid, anhydrous ammonia, drain cleaner, rubbing alcohol, gasoline, antifreeze and/or lantern fuel along with other poisonous and corrosive cleaning products. Manufacturers secure in their market share will often cut their meth, but new or opportunistic meth makers might attract customers with the purest product possible. But purity is an elusive goal and the bonding and activating agents virtually always make their way into the finished product. Every dose of meth includes the ingestion of some unknown agent. More often than not, meth users are unwittingly dropping laxatives in their coffee, snorting lye up their noses, smoking gasoline or injecting battery acid into their veins.

The overwhelming majority of the poisons used to make meth, however, generally end up being dumped. This puts a remarkable amount of toxic waste into our shared environment. Estimates put the ratio of waste to product for the process at about six to one, meaning that for every pound of meth made, about six pounds of waste chemicals are dumped into our soil, streams and sewers. It's a quantity of toxic output that would have a factory closed immediately and its owner jailed. Making matters worse is the fact that a great deal of meth is made on environmentally sensitive lands—like national forests. Not all of the pollution goes down into the land and water. Most rural meth makers get rid of much of their lab waste by making "burn piles"—collections of all the empty cold-pill boxes, lye bottles and other containers that held the raw materials used in the process which are set alight. The raw and usually extremely toxic smoke billows into the sky completely unfiltered.

But all of these problems can occur only if the cook actually survives the dangerous production process. Cooking meth isn't easy. It involves a number of procedures involving poisonous, caustic, flammable and even explosive ingredients. One wrong move, one cut corner and boom! And, frankly, not all meth cooks have a reputation for being all that smart or careful. At a March 2005 conference for politicians, doctors, police and social workers in Tennessee, there was a mandatory stop at the burn ward at the Vanderbilt University Medical Center. Seven of the twenty patients there at the time were being treated for meth lab-related injuries.

"As bad as this may sound, as a burn doctor I almost wish another drug—one less volatile that doesn't regularly explode during the manufacturing process—would come down the pike to overtake the popularity of meth," says Dr. Jeff Guy, the center's director. He introduced attendees to a patient. The man had no medical insurance and had been severely burned in an explosion while manufacturing meth. The patient needed to stay in the burn ward for forty-five days at a cost of about $240,000. When informed the patient was receiving a government disability check every month, one of the politicians pointed out that the man appeared to be severely injured and in no condition to be released.

Guy replied that he was talking about another incident with the same man last October. Upon his first release, Guy said, he went back to his lab and "gone out and blown himself up again."

The number of meth-related burn victims Guy has seen is still climbing. Worse, he said, were the increasing numbers of children who have been burned by fires or explosions, innocent victims, he suspects, of cooks operating at-home meth labs.

ONCE KNOWN AS "America's hometown," Hannibal, Missouri was the home of popular storyteller and satirist Mark Twain. The town of eighteen thousand situated on the banks of the Mississippi has fallen on hard times, and has a reported crime rate more than double that of the national average. Those statistics put it up with some of America's largest cities, many of which have improved their crime rates significantly as crack use has waned.

Hannibal police chief Lyndell Davis is doing her best, but is resigned to the fact that petty crime occurs with depressing frequency.

"Mark Twain Avenue—it's like the flip of a quarter to see which one they hit next," she said, referring to the strip of fast food outlets and convenience stores where many robberies, break-ins and muggings occur.

"It's getting crazy," said one long-time Hannibal resident I spoke with. "The place is overrun by crime. It's been that way ever since the meth showed up."

While lots of places consider themselves the worst hit by meth, only one has the dubious honor of official sanctioning. According to Republican senator Kit Bond:

Located in the middle of the country, with many small towns, national forest acres, the rural makeup and the number of interstate highways, Missouri is a draw for methamphetamine cookers, distributors, dealers and smugglers. In recent years Missouri has become known as the 'meth capital' of the United States.

And Missouri has been hit hard. According to Morgan Quitno Press, a Lawrence, Kansas-based research firm which compiled the list using statistics from the FBI and local police forces, St. Louis (after years of coming close) has finally knocked Detroit off the top of the list of most dangerous places to live in the United States. St. Louis, the biggest city is Missouri, is particularly affected by crimes such as car theft, robbery, break-ins and domestic disputes, which are all often related to meth. In 2006, the FBI reported an increase in the overall crime rate in the U.S.—the first after thirteen straight years of decline. According to a CNN report, "crime increased most noticeably in several categories in many mid-sized cities and in the Midwest."

It's an area that's becoming something of a meth belt.

The story is much the same in Canada. While conventional wisdom would probably predict that the highest crime rates would be found in huge population centers like Toronto and Montreal or in traditionally tough mill towns like Hamilton or Sherbrooke, they actually occur farther west. Not surprisingly, in towns and cities hit hard by meth. According to Statistics Canada, the six cities of 100,000 or more residents with the highest crime rates in 2004 were Regina, Saskatoon, Abbotsford, Winnipeg, Vancouver and Edmonton. Except for Vancouver, which has a long history of drug-related crime, all are relatively new to the top of the list. And all of them have serious meth problems. Edmonton, which saw its arrests for meth possession jump from six to 279 in one year, is sometimes slightingly referred to as "Methmonton."

WHO WOULDN'T
WANT BETTER SEX?

EVERYTHING YOU NEED TO know about why
people take meth can be summed up in a quote by one of its
most ardent and vociferous enemies. Paul Laymon, assistant
U.S. attorney for Chattanooga, Tennessee, and an expert at prosecuting meth cases, described its allure to a collection of cops
and lawyers.

"Who wouldn't want to use it?" he asked rhetorically. "You
lose weight and you have great sex."

He's right. Meth can supply almost perfect happiness—at
least at first.

I CAN TELL FROM THE second he walks into the cof-
fee shop that he's the guy. I can also tell that we probably won't
like each other very much. Nothing particular, just a vibe. But I
wave and he comes over. Brian's in his late thirties, but he looks
quite a bit older. He's about my height and maybe two-thirds my
weight. He has closely cropped gray hair and a soul patch. He's

wearing a Che Guevara T-shirt tucked into his shorts and one of those godawful Tilley hats. The overall effect makes him look far geekier than I expected. He sits and, after a few pleasantries, I ask him what he wants. I go up to the counter and bring back a tall Americano for me and a caramel latte with hazelnut syrup for him.

We stare across the table at each other and I'm totally at a loss for something to say. I normally try to break the ice in tense situations by saying something unexpected or provocative. We're in a coffee shop not far from the center of Toronto's gay village and I stand out a bit as an obviously straight guy, so I thought I'd play on that.

"It's funny, y'know," I said to him. "When I'm in a straight bar, nobody pays attention to me. But when I'm in a gay bar, I get hit on constantly."

He looked me up and down and paused. "Well, the things that make you less attractive to women actually work in your favor with some men in the gay community," he said. "Your wedding ring says that you're interested in quick anonymous sex without any strings, and the extra weight you're carrying around your midsection tells me that you don't have any frightening diseases or serious drug habits."

He may not like me, but it looks like he'll talk—and be honest and frank.

In Brian's defense, he really didn't want to talk to me anyway. I was discussing meth with some people I knew at my sons' school and one of them took me aside and said I should speak with her cousin. A few days later, she introduced me to Carlos, a twenty-five-year-old who rarely stops talking and never seems to stop moving. He was happy to see me because he wanted someone to talk some sense into his boyfriend, Brian. They'd been going out for a while and there was some talk of moving in together, but Carlos (whose boundless energy seems to be entirely natural) wouldn't make any commitments until Brian stopped using meth. Actually, he confided in me, it would probably be okay if Brian used it a little bit on the sly, but at least told him he'd quit.

I could tell Carlos was sincerely worried. He'd been hanging around the club scene since he was a teenager and he'd seen what meth could do. "Some guys, you know, they take the meth and, at first, it's great," he told me. "They have a good time and stay hard all night—that's important for the older guys—but if they keep doing it, it makes them stupid." And he definitely didn't want to see Brian, who it was clear he sincerely cared for, get stupid.

Talking to Carlos actually makes me feel a bit guilty. I can't really help Brian. I'm talking to him for my own selfish reasons. I'm writing a book about meth and I need to know more—every user I talk to teaches me another story, another few words and a better understanding of the subject. To tell the truth, a year ago, I didn't know much more about meth than most people. But while I was researching *Fellen Angels*, I came across it over and over again. I saw how much it had become part of our society and the colossal amount of damage it could do. I saw it, I was there. Meth users were at the bottom of the evolutionary ladder of all the people I met in that world. They were the most addicted, the most desperate, the most willing to do anything for another ten bucks and, by far, the most pathetic. The dealers knew it and they didn't care.

As I look across the table from Brian, I know I can't help him. I can't say anything he hasn't heard a million times before and already shut out in favor of what he gets from meth. All I can do is find out more.

"So," I say. "Tell me about the high."

"What? You're writing a book about meth and you haven't even tried it?" he snorts. "That's ridiculous."

He's got a point, actually. And I was going to try it; after all, what's one hit? Well, according to a survey of experts from groups like the World Health Organization, the National Institute on Drug Abuse (NIDA) and the American Medical Association conducted by Philip J. Hilts of *The New York Times*, one hit could actually be enough. On a scale of 0 to 100 (with a higher number meaning more addictive) crystal meth scored 93, heroin 80, cocaine 72 and marijuana 21. The numbers published by the U.S. government's Drug Enforcement Agency (DEA) are even more startling. Crystal meth scores a 98 on their scale, while nothing else (not even crack) breaks the 80 mark. According to their literature, the DEA says that the number corresponds to the percentage of people who are addicted to the drug a year after first trying it. While many may scoff at the idea of 98 percent of first-time meth users hooked a year later and attribute it to the DEA's overzealous attempts to scare people away from drugs, it doesn't explain why crack, heroin, PCP, marijuana and all the other drugs the DEA is trying to combat got off so easily in comparison. While there's an argument to be made that the DEA's numbers are inflated, it's harder to debate the order they've been put in.

According to the doctors I've spoken with, meth does far more damage to the brain than any of the other commonly used drugs and much of it just can't ever be repaired. According to NIDA, a branch of the U.S. government's National Institute of Health, "research has also shown that meth can cause a variety of cardiovascular problems, including rapid heart rate, irregular heartbeat, increased blood pressure, and irreversible, stroke-producing damage to small blood vessels in the brain. Hyperthermia (elevated body temperature) and convulsions occur with meth overdoses and, if not treated immediately, can result in death." Those aren't the things that happen to the long-term addict, those are actually the potential side effects of a routine high.

Those who defend meth (and there are a surprising number who do, mostly on civil liberties grounds) are quick to point out that very few people die of meth overdose—certainly far fewer than from cocaine or heroin.

"Oh, they don't die from overdose," says Sgt. Jerome Engele, head of the Integrated Drug Unit for the Saskatoon police. "They die from the hallucinations or suicide that comes with the depression after the drug wears off. We had a young woman here who walked in front of a speeding car on Christmas Day when she was coming down."

Suicides aren't that rare.

"Users commonly experience a number of psychotic features, including paranoia, auditory hallucinations, mood disturbances, and delusions," says UCLA's Rawson. "The paranoia can result in homicidal as well as suicidal thoughts."

But all drug users know that the Darwin factor always takes a few, no matter what the drug. There are always people who'll use too much, too often or the drug they are taking will simply be the wrong one, the one that triggers in them a response that isn't right, isn't logical and could well end up with them on a cold metal slab in the coroner's office. Death isn't much of a deterrent to a meth addict, because everyone thinks it won't happen to them, and most of them are right. But living with the cumulative effects of meth addiction isn't always preferable to dying from them.

According to NIDA, "methamphetamine abusers exhibit symptoms that can include violent behavior, anxiety, depression, confusion and insomnia. They also can display a number of psychotic features, including paranoia, auditory hallucinations and delusions."

It's not just the doctors and the narcs that preach abstinence. I have met lots of drug users and even dealers who have no interest in meth. It's not the penalties associated with trafficking the stuff; it's the guilt. A street-level dealer I know in Montreal (where the meth trade is still small but growing, especially among the gay community) refuses to carry it, despite the huge profits.

"It's bad stuff," he told me. "People smoke marijuana and they get happy; people smoke that stuff and they go nuts."

I've even talked to crack addicts—people many of us think have already thrown their lives away—and they won't even go near meth.

It's not the numbers and the scary stats that kept me from taking that first hit of meth. It's the base, instinctive knowledge that I'd like it too much to ever stop. So I admit to Brian that I don't have the guts. That makes him pretty happy. He's a bit more confident now and he asks me if I want to see what it's like. Of course, I tell him I do. He tells me to wait and heads into the men's room.

START WITH A HAZMAT SUIT

The government of Oklahoma has prepared the following guidelines for land owners who attempt to clean up meth labs on their property.

1. Determine if the property was used for meth production.
2. Air out the property before and during cleanup.
3. Before entering the property to clean, put on personal protective equipment such as gloves, protective clothing and eye protection. Respirators that offer protection against vapors are recommended.
4. Remove all unnecessary items and dispose of them properly.
5. Remove all visibly contaminated items or items that have an odor.
6. Clean all surfaces using proper household cleaning methods and proper personal protection.
7. Clean the ventilation system.
8. Leave plumbing cleanup to the experts.
9. Air out the property for three to five days.
10. If odor or staining remains, have your home evaluated by a professional.
11. Dispose of clothing, gloves, brushes and rags used during the cleaning process.
12. Review additional guidance on personal decontamination provided by local law enforcement.

Source: Oklahoma Department of Environmental Quality

He comes out about fifteen minutes later. I'm not kidding, it was only fifteen minutes, but he came out a changed man. Seriously, this nothing of a man who was in front of me earlier returned full of vitality. He had better color in his face and I'll be damned if he didn't appear at least twenty pounds heavier. He was smiling, almost laughing. It was a different man who sat across the table from me now. He was still fiddling with things, but now it was like he was discovering them for the first time. The world appeared to be full of endless fascination for him. Hell, he even liked me.

He was grinning cockily from ear to ear. He seemed to radiate accomplishment. I ask him what it's like, what he's going through right now.

"It's absolutely orgasmic," he says. "That's the only word I have for it—orgasmic."

That's a pretty commonly used metaphor. Pretty much every time I've spoken to a meth user, the word "orgasm"—or some variation—is used to describe the high.

A cop told me about a nineteen-year-old girl who asked him if he'd ever had a "climax." He told her he had. "Well, meth is like ten of those all at once. That's why I can't stop."

While I'll admit Brian looks pretty happy, he hardly looks to be in the throes of an orgasm. I tell him that. He laughs.

"Well, I spent the best part of it in there," he said, referring to the men's room. There is, he tells me, two different highs from meth. The first, which only lasts a few minutes, is exhilarating. As the hormones that meth triggers wash through the bloodstream, every part of the body feels the rush.

"It's massive," Brian tells me. "It flows through your body like Niagara Falls. I can even hear it bubbling up through my ears on its way to my brain."

Actually, it's already been to his brain and is headed in the other direction. What Brian hears in his ears is actually an increase in his heart rate and blood pressure. The blood vessels in his ears were handling extra flow, and that was what he was hearing.

But after spending a few minutes with Brian, I don't see any actual joy. Certainly, he looks better than he did before he went into the mens' room, but he's far from ecstasy. So I ask him, if meth is so great, how come he only looks okay. "Oh, I used to get that way," he tells me. "But I've been taking it for a while and I guess I've built up something of an immunity." Although the highs he's been getting have been steadily weakening, he's too scared, he said, to increase his dosage.

About four months ago, Brian was, by his own admission, feeling old. He was going to clubs and getting tired long before the pairing off began. And, he tells me, that he wasn't performing the way he had when he was younger. He tried to buy Viagra off the Internet and wound up, as most do, humiliated and poorer for the experience. But then he found out about meth. The guy who introduced him to it, free of charge, told him it'd solve all of his problems.

It did.

After his first hit, he thought he was coming for a half hour. But he was surprised to discover that he was still hard. For the next six hours.

He had everything he wanted. He had more energy, he didn't need to sleep or eat, he was losing weight and his dick was working like it did a dozen years ago, only better. He wanted more.

That's about when he met Carlos. He was pretty sure he was in love and he wanted to make certain that he was the man that Carlos had fallen for, not the man he was before he started taking meth.

"Before I started taking meth, I was bored, lonely and fat," he told me. "Now I have an excellent lover, I'm thin and I'm happy." It's pretty hard to argue with results like that.

I asked him if he smoked in the washroom.

"No, too risky," he said. "People go nuts if they smell smoke in any establishment now. Smoking's illegal everywhere these days and someone will chase you down, even in a stall, to stop you. It gets a bit embarrassing when what you're smoking is illegal." Besides, he says, he tends to cough when he smokes anything, even through a bong. Instead, he usually snorts meth like cocaine. To demonstrate, he pulls a little metal and glass cylinder about the size of a spark plug out of his pocket and hands it to me. "It's called a bullet," he says. "You fill it with the flakes, shake it up, put it under your nostril and—pow!—a perfectly metered dose every time."

I ask him if he's worried about having it out at the coffee shop. He laughs.

"Anybody who knows what it is won't care," he said. "Besides, bullets aren't illegal; you can buy them at the head shops up and down Yonge Street or on the Internet." He says he usually gets high by snorting, but it can irritate his nose, especially if he hasn't ground the meth chips into a fine enough powder. When his nose is acting up, he dumps the meth in a beverage and takes it that way. "It's okay, but it takes forever to get high," he said. "And it's not nearly as intense." I asked him what "forever" means.

"About twenty minutes."

When I ask him about needles, he says that's where he draws the line.

"I'd never do that," he said. "Those guys expose themselves to so many injuries and diseases, plus you have to keep getting new needles, it's just too much." While he doesn't exactly scoff at needle users, or "pricks" as he calls them, he does indicate that he considers them perhaps a bit more addicted, somewhat more desperate than people like him.

While the bulk of Brian's meth goes up his nose, that's not actually his favorite method. He begins to tell me about "booty bumping," which is when the meth is dissolved in water then inserted into the anus (usually by a partner) and absorbed through the rectal membranes like a suppository. It was at this very moment I first noticed how loudly he was talking. I asked him why it was a better high—was it quicker or more intense?

"Not really, but it's more localized," he said. There are extra dangers associated with the practice, though. The rectal membranes are even more fragile than those in the nose and big chunks of meth can be abrasive and cause irritation or internal bleeding. He assured me sex while booty bumping was the most pleasurable sensation he'd ever experienced. I told him I'd have to take his word for it. He started laughing uproariously at that predictable little half-joke and I began to take stock of how animated he was. He really was a different person than the guy who'd walked in. He was confident, gregarious, talkative and interesting, if a bit annoying.

It's not just men who indulge meth in the hopes of better and more intense sex. Taylor, who goes by a different name when she poses nude on the website her ex-boyfriend set up for her, or when she occasionally dances in strip clubs when she needs money, has been using meth for a few months now and says that it gets her in the mood.

"I usually take meth when I'm going out to a club, so I can stay up all night," she says. "But it always seems to affect me that way." She tells me that when she takes meth her libido accelerates for hours afterwards. "Maybe it's the excess energy," she laughs. "I just don't know what to do with myself—it's a good thing I'm single again."

DR. MARY HOLLEY, an Alabama-based obstetrician, became an anti-meth activist after her addicted brother committed suicide. In her book *They Call it Ice*, she writes about treating a teenage girl who, on a meth binge, contracted five different sexually transmitted diseases from five different partners in a single night.

Meth does a lot of things besides inflating one's sex drive. When high, meth users have more energy, a heightened sense of self-esteem and confidence, they don't need to eat as much (which, along with the extra energy, leads to rapid weight loss) or sleep, and they experience a clarity of thought that allows them to make decisions more quickly and firmly.

Because of these qualities, many users take a hit before work, especially if they have high-stress positions. Entertainers, doctors, Wall Street brokers, even athletes.

In his classic 1970 book *Ball Four*, major-league pitcher Jim Bouton wrote that amphetamine use was rampant in the high-stakes, performance-oriented world of professional baseball.

Amphetamine, as the name implies, is a lot like methamphetamine. The forerunner of meth, amphetamine is chemically similar and has the same effects, but in a much smaller magnitude. Called "greenies" by most players, amphetamines were accepted as part of the business by many players, but rarely talked about. "How fabulous are greenies?" Bouton wrote. "Some of the guys have to take one just to get their hearts to start beating." Most clubhouses, he said, had two coffee pots: "leaded," which had amphetamines, and "unleaded," which didn't.

Jim Leyritz was a backup catcher who spent most of his career with the Yankees, but later bounced around with the Angels, Rangers, Padres, Red Sox and Dodgers as his skills declined. Although he's best known for a home run he hit against the Braves in the 1996 World Series that helped the Yankees establish a dynasty, Leyritz was a career light hitter, even for a backup.

In an interview on a nationally syndicated radio show in January 2006, Leyritz admitted his own greenie use. In his

SIGNS OF ABUSE

Although many of the symptoms of meth abuse are internal, there are indicators that indicate someone is a frequent user:

- Anxiety
- Depression
- Elevated body temperature
- Fiddling, twitching and other seemingly involuntary motions
- Increased blood pressure

- Infections and sores at injection sites
- Insomnia
- Irritability
- Lack of appetite and weight loss
- Nausea, vomiting and diarrhea
- Paranoia

- Red, sore and runny noses
- Seizures
- Skin ulceration and infection

Source: Personal interviews, various published reports

rookie year, he said, some teammates took him out drinking and he showed up at the clubhouse the following day with a raging hangover. He was shocked to learn he would be starting at catcher in that day's game. Since he could barely stand up, let alone withstand the rigors of playing the toughest position in the game, and he knew his still-tenuous hold on a major-league job hung in the balance, Leyritz drank the "leaded" coffee. That day, he recorded three hits in four at-bats, including two home runs. Over a career that lasted eleven seasons, he claimed he never used amphetamines again.

Although amphetamines have long been illegal without a prescription, they weren't banned or tested for by Major League Baseball (or the National Football League) until the 2006 season. While the news of baseball's ban made few headlines in an era when the sport is rarely mentioned without the word "steroids" along with it, the players certainly noticed.

"Steroids are not the problem," said a well-known veteran baseball player who insisted on anonymity. "They got the wrong one. I don't even know anybody who used steroids. Everybody uses amphetamines." And those that do, will certainly miss them.

"There are days you just have to have it," added another regular. "When you have that bad travel day and you've got to be at the field early in the morning, it's tough."

NASTY STUFF

Anhydrous ammonia, a key ingredient in some methods of meth manufacture, can damage human tissue in a variety of ways. Since the chemical is largely unavailable to clandestine chemists, it often has to be stolen, resulting in leaks, explosions and spills.

Dehydration: Anhydrous ammonia will dehydrate body tissue. Contact of the liquid or vapors with the eyes will result in serious injury or blindness. Any tissue contact with the liquid will cause first-, second- and third-degree burns. Acute exposure to vapors will bring about lung damage and possible suffocation.

Caustic burning: Anhydrous ammonia in combination with water extracted from body tissue creates a strong base that further damages body tissue by chemical burning.

Freezing: When liquid anhydrous ammonia vaporizes, it pulls heat from its surroundings. Body tissue exposed to liquid anhydrous ammonia will freeze almost instantly.

Source: Minnesota Department of Public Safety

AFTER THE HIGH:
THE FALLOUT

KYLE PROBABLY WOULDN'T like Brian very much. He almost certainly has no idea what booty bumping is. But he has something in common with Brian: meth.

Brian is gay, urban and the manager of a gourmet foods retail store; Kyle is straight, semirural and a self-employed "largely under the table" contractor and landscaper. He's never heard of Che Guevara (I checked) and tends to wear T-shirts with snappy, though not entirely witty, sayings on them or the names of bars or other places he's visited or would like to. He also likes to add various baseball caps as accents.

I meet with Kyle in a dreary doughnut shop. He is thin, like Brian, but much younger and with none of his studied and affected polish. He seems like a nice enough guy and, unlike his urban counterpart, he arrives upbeat and smiling. I correctly surmise that he's already taken meth earlier that day. It's hot out and his job is tough. He is doing lawn and garden upkeep for a local business and that means a lot of hard, sweaty and tedious work. The woman who hired him is something of a hardass and he knows she will be watching him every minute he is there. If he wants more work, he'll have to impress her. In a small town, the opinion of an influential businesswoman can mean the difference between success and failure.

Not surprisingly, Kyle was introduced to meth at work. Before he went into business for himself, Kyle worked for a guy named Jim. Jim used to show up early for every job, he worked hard and expected the boys on his crew to do the same.

"Working for Jim was a real eye-opener," Kyle tells me. "There was no sitting around with him; if you expected to be paid, you had to work for it." A week into the job, when Kyle was pretty sure he was going to quit or be fired, one of the better workers introduced him to meth.

"Robbie came up to me and told me that everyone was talking about how I was in trouble," he says. "Then he told me that everyone else was using meth." Faced with the threat of losing his job, Kyle got desperate. "So I decided to give it a try. Robbie set me up with my first hit," he says. "And, well, I loved it."

Kyle downplays the sexual aspect of meth, but he practically sounds like a commercial for the stuff on other grounds. I ask him about the rush.

"It kinda floods over you, just like that, yeah, it flows upward, like you're being dipped in water," he tells me. "But it's not like water, it's like a cold shot of something, something really, really good." When describing the meth high, Kyle uses a lot of words like "good," "great" and "excellent." He's not really very descriptive, but he tries. I push him to be more specific. "It's kind of like, well, think of the best day of your life," he said. "It's like that all day, every day." I asked him what he meant by that. He was growing frustrated by this point, and he told me: "It's impossible for you to know what it feels like unless you try it."

A LITTLE MORE THAN a week later, I was actually surprised to get Kyle at home because he rarely answers the phone. When I called, intending just to leave another message, his mother answered. She was over there taking care of him. "Seems he's got a touch of the flu and he can't go into work today," she told me. I asked if I could talk to him and she said she'd check to see if he was awake. When he got on the phone, he sounded awful. In a labored, scratchy voice, he asked, "Can I call you back in about an hour?" I knew that he was willing to talk to me, but not in front of his mom.

About ninety minutes later I called him back. I could tell from his response that I'd woke him, even though it was four in the afternoon. I told him I didn't want to bother him if he was sick. "Not sick," he admitted. "Hungover." He and some friends went out the night before for some guy's bachelor party and Kyle ended up doing some meth. "They had strippers there and everyone was really having a good time," he said. "I don't think I got home until five." He wasn't just drinking, he was taking meth. He had stayed awake for a couple of days. "Actually, I only had two beers and I didn't even finish the second one—I don't like to mix alcohol and meth," he said. "I would go outside to smoke."

I asked him if a meth hangover was anything like an alcohol hangover. "Kind of, but not really," he said in that annoyingly obtuse way of his. "You don't get sick to your stomach, but the headache is worse and you feel bad for a lot longer." How long depends on how much you've taken and how long you've been using. I've had people, especially those bingeing on large quantities of meth, tell me that they've had hangovers for up to four days. The most frequently reported effects include, fever, chills, an inability to eat, headache, confusion, hallucinations, anger, torpor and mind-bending depression.

One of the big differences between meth and alcohol is that when you wake up after being high on meth, you remember every little thing that happened the night before, often in horrible, crystal-clear detail. And, all speed users, especially meth users, have a hard-won reputation as being unpredictable, antisocial and sometimes violent.

"Abusers of amphetamine are prone to accidents because the drug produces excitation and grandiosity followed by excess fatigue and sleeplessness," reads an entry in *The Merck Manual*, an encyclopedia of pharmaceuticals and their effects, which is frequently consulted by physicians. "Amphetamine abuse may lead to serious antisocial behavior and can precipitate a schizophrenic episode." Amphetamine, after all, is an extremely low-octane relative of methamphetamine. Prolonged meth use—known as "tweaking"—is defined by the University of Maryland's Center for Substance Abuse Research (CESAR), as:

> A dangerous stage of meth abuse that occurs when an abuser who has not slept in three to fifteen days becomes irritable and paranoid. The tweaker craves more meth but finds it difficult to achieve the original high, causing frustration and unpredictable behavior. Such behavior can turn violent, leading to impulsive criminal behavior, domestic disputes or motor vehicle accidents.

I asked Kyle if he'd ever done anything he regrets while high on meth. "Sure, lots of times, but my friends do lots of the same kinds of things when they're drunk," he said. He won't go into any kind of detail, but he'll admit to some light vandalism and something he calls "freaking with people." From his description, it sounds like he's strangely proud of his hobby of scaring passersby. "I love it when a car's stopped at a stoplight and it's the middle of the night," he said, beginning to sound much more animated that he did a few minutes earlier. "I come running out of the bushes and grab the door handle and start pulling—you should see the look on people's faces; I think half of them probably wet their pants."

Like many meth users, Kyle takes the edge off his hangover with marijuana. "Oh yeah, without a joint or two I'd go crazy," he said. "It doesn't make the hangover go away, but it sure does help." But it also presents him with a bit of a problem. While the weed calms him down, it also puts him to sleep. Since meth, a natural anti-somniac, keeps you awake all night, the crash afterwards is huge. Not only have you missed a night's sleep, but you were probably hyperactive while you were doing it. Once the meth is metabolized, your body is going to want the sleep it feels you owe it, and perhaps more. Adding marijuana to the mix only makes it worse. Kyle was grateful that the party was on a Wednesday night because it gave him time to recuperate before work again on Monday.

Taylor's experiences with meth hangovers are a bit different. "Really, it just makes me sad," she said. "It's a terrible feeling. And it's not just the hangover. It's the guilt that goes along with it." Meth has gotten rather routine for her. The highs aren't very high and the lows are much lower and longer than they had been. Unlike Kyle, who takes a little weed to assuage his hangover, Taylor either waits it out or takes a little more meth. "I'll just use a little and only if I'm *really* hungover," she said. "I don't want to become addicted." Luckily, she only works when she wants to. She can do a weekend photo shoot which will keep her website going for a few months, she chats online with her most devoted fans every few weeks or so. And she dances whenever she feels she needs the money. She doesn't like dancing, but loves the freedom of making her own hours. "I guess you could say I work on meth and I work for meth," she laughed unconvincingly.

When I ask her to describe a meth hangover, she's not much more help than Kyle. "It sucks, I can tell you that," she said.

WORSE THAN HEROIN?

The following was posted as a comment to a story about meth hysteria on talkleft.org:

Well, I can't speak for anyone else, but my wife is a Portland social worker who works with homeless youth, and she says there's no bigger obstacle to her clients' welfare than meth. She'd rather they get hooked on heroin than meth, because her clients have been more successful kicking heroin. And she has no love for the effects of meth on her kids. She's counseled a number of clients who appear to have permanently damaged their circuits from overusing the drug.

Would she call it a crisis? I don't know. But I'm sure she wouldn't dismiss the idea or claim that it's not a problem. She says it's an ugly drug, and I think she'd laugh at anyone who tried to compare it to garden-variety speed.

Source: talkleft.org

I ask her about her behavior when high and what she regretted doing. "It's not 'what' I regret, it's who," she said with a chuckle. Then she told me something that surprised me. "I'm usually pretty under control when I'm high," she said. "But it's different when I'm really hungover—it was so bad a couple of times I tried to kill myself." Her attempts weren't really very serious. On one, she swallowed a bottle of anti-nausea pills and called her ex-boyfriend. A quick trip to the hospital and she was better in two days. A few weeks later, she drove his car into a ditch, but sustained only a few minor cuts and bruises. "I thought it'd roll," she told me. "I guess I wasn't going fast enough." She laughs it off now, explaining that she's matured a great deal in the last few months and says she realizes that the self-loathing and the depression are chemical aspects of the hangover, not how she actually feels about herself.

Actually, meth-related suicides are pretty commonplace. Officials in Montana and other states report that their suicide rates have shot up remarkably since meth arrived in force. One Iowa cop I spoke with told me that whenever his department comes across the body of a young person, they assume the cause is meth-related suicide. And, if the body is that of a thin young person, they're sure of it. The problem isn't just that meth users are depressed or that they envision a bleak world of endless money-draining and health-sapping addiction in front of them. While that may be true and enough to spur thoughts of suicide, many doctors believe that withdrawal from meth use—even the amount caused by a hangover—can actually cause chemical reactions in the brain that prevent the suppression of suicidal thoughts. Those thoughts are a normal byproduct of brain activity, but are normally kept under control by brain chemicals that are scarce or absent during a meth hangover.

Brian told me, however, he never, ever thinks about suicide. "Homicide maybe, but not suicide," he jokes. He credits his lack of suicidal thoughts to his close friends, primarily Carlos. "Without him, I'd be an absolute mess," he said. "He provides the grounding I need to stay sane."

So I spoke again with Carlos, who originally came to me because he was concerned about Brian's meth use.

"Of course I love him, but when he has too much meth, he can turn into a real jerk, you know, like a bully," he tells me. "I know he has a lot of pent-up frustration in him—his parents, old relationships—and it all comes out at me when he's high. I know it's not meant for me, but it's pretty hard for anybody to put up with that much abuse." I asked him if Brian ever got physically abusive when he was high, and Carlos demurs.

"What about when he's hungover?" I ask him.

"Oh, he's just a big grouch," he replies. "Not abusive, just nasty."

ARE WE ALL ADDICTED TO SOMETHING? A BRIEF HISTORY

I CAN BARELY GO TO my brother's house without getting drunk.

You'd think we'd know better—our parents were alcoholics—but we persist, as long as our kids aren't there and we're not driving. We drink and drink and drink and generally lose track of how much. We're not angry drunks, so we always have a good time, although I'm not sure the other people around us always do.

Perhaps it's cultural. While alcohol use occurs in virtually every society with varying degrees of acceptance, it's almost mandatory in ours. As the sons of generations of Scottish, English and Irish drinkers, it's in our blood. Alcohol has been thoroughly entrenched in European cultures for thousands of years and nowhere is it more deeply embedded than the British Isles. And it's been faithfully carried on in their North American descendants. We drink when we're happy (weddings, parties); we drink when we're sad (funerals, wakes). We regard our children's first time coming home drunk as a time-honored rite of passage. When my own parents caught me walking down the street with a case of twenty-four bottles of cheap, domestic beer proudly swung over my shoulder when I was fifteen, they laughed, confiscated the booty and drank it themselves. Many of us regard an ability to consume vast amounts of alcohol to be equivalent to manliness. Few of us haven't been told about how children and even infants were given Guinness during the blitz because it was the most nutritious thing available, and my family and my peers generally considered people who didn't drink as strange and even potentially dangerous. There's a *Saturday Night Live* sketch from 1993 in which Mike Myers, who's of Scottish descent but was playing a Jewish character based loosely on his mother-in-law, said of an Irish character played by Charlton Heston: "Get him a bowl of whiskey, that's what these people are like."

Trust me, we are.

It's not just the British and Irish. French and Italian kids, we're told, enjoy wine with lunch and dinner as soon as they're taking solid food. Beer originated in Central Europe and is almost religiously celebrated and revered there and pretty much everywhere else. Munich's Oktoberfest may well be the world's largest festival, drawing six million visitors every year. While it originated as a celebration of the fall harvest, it's pretty much all about the beer now. The Scandinavians are big drinkers and so are the Spaniards and Portuguese. The Greeks have ouzo and the Balkan nations are famous for slivovitz and other brandies. And no people, not even the Irish, are reputed to drink as much as the Russians. Hell, even our common religion, Christianity, demands we drink wine as part of the holy sacrament. As with their languages, religious beliefs and other customs, Europeans have exported alcohol and its use all over the world. There are few countries where you can't buy a beer or a glass of wine, generally only those with strict Islamic governments. And even there, there are usually ways around it for important visitors and savvy locals.

And, despite the cost of this highly taxed hobby, despite the beer bellies, the dead brain cells, the violence and the traffic accidents and the potential diseases and all the other drawbacks, we keep on drinking. We do it because we like it. It feels good. It makes us confident, happy and bold. It allows us to overcome our natural shyness and say and do things we normally wouldn't have the courage to. How many of us can say we lost our virginity, proposed marriage, got married or celebrated any important occasion without the help of the demon drink? It unites us and generally just makes us happy. It's addictive and, for the most part, we don't care.

But no drinker enjoys what happens after the buzz wears off. Hangovers are the natural and predictable consequence of drinking, but we always seem to forget about them while we're earning them. Those who haven't suffered a hangover simply don't have the ability to conceive of the horrible torment one causes. An intense, insistent headache that won't allow you to stay still, but hurts worse when you move, is combined with a gut-clearing nausea, a hypersensitivity to light and especially noise, aches and pains in every muscle and joint, an inability to concentrate and an overwhelmingly bad mood.

There are all kinds of folk remedy cures and diet supplements that claim to prevent them, but they don't really work.

"I have never found any panacea for a hangover," said seventeenth-century English philosopher and noted alcohol enthusiast Francis Bacon. "I don't think one exists apart from suicide."

Sadly, the science of the "morning after" hasn't really progressed much. "No compelling evidence exists to suggest that any conventional or complementary intervention is effective for preventing or treating alcohol hangover," writes Dr. Max Pittler of Exeter University in *The British Medical Journal.* "The most effective way to avoid the symptoms of alcohol induced hangover is to practice abstinence or moderation."

But every drinker knows the doctor is wrong. There is one sure cure for a hangover and that's another drink. Commonly referred to as a "hair o' the dog that bit you" (derived from an old Scottish saying about the joy of revenge) a next-morning drink can ease or eliminate the symptoms of a hangover—if you can keep it down. But it also presents a stark precipice, the other side of which may be a rapid and irrevocable slide into alcohol dependency. We all know it's addictive and we've all seen what it can do. Walk down a major thoroughfare of any large city and you'll see the victims of alcohol addiction. You've seen them, gaunt, filthy and desperate—begging for money they often say will go to food but you probably can't help thinking will be spent on more alcohol. If you're drinking to offset the ill effects of earlier drinking, you're getting dangerously close to having to drink all the time just to stave off the hangovers. We all know it's possible that the next drink you have could be a step on a voyage that may end with you on a street corner shaking an old coffee cup at passersby and saving their change until you can scrounge enough for a forty-ounce bottle of malt liquor. Although it's not often a stirring enough image to make many people stop drinking, it's usually sufficiently powerful to make most of us limit our alcohol intake to evenings and social events.

It's too late for abstinence or moderation for me. I got drunk last night and I have a hangover as I write this. Years of practice have taught me what's good for me. I need food, preferably greasy, something to drink, and caffeine. I choose Diet Coke over coffee because the carbonation delivers the caffeine to my system quicker and coffee's a diuretic—not suitable at a time when my body needs fluids. People often say carbonated beverages are diuretics too, but my body knows better and it's right. The urban legend grew out of the fact that most soft drinks contain caffeine and the chemical is itself a small-bore diuretic. But that caffeine is surrounded by an overwhelming amount of water.

"The amount of diuretic in Coke is not enough to get rid of all the fluid that's in the drink," says Charles Hensley, Ph.D., and CEO of PRB Pharmaceuticals, a major pharmaceuticals research and development firm. Coke may be slightly less hydrating than pure water because of the caffeine, but it may actually be better for those in the unholy throes of a hangover. "You don't always want to drink water when you're hungover," Hensley said. "Your body is craving sugary beverages because the sugar helps energize receptors that transport water into your body." So Coke is actually more effective than water for quick hydration—the caffeine's just a bonus.

While caffeine does nothing to cure the more pressing symptoms of a hangover, it will give me back a little bit of energy and help me think straight. Caffeine may not be a cure for my chronic minor alcohol overdoses, but it does sort of act as its opposite. Alcohol is technically a depressant, but that's a misleading term. It actually makes us happy by turning on some of the hormones that put us to sleep, so the "depression" we feel is actually a putting to sleep of many of the fears, inhibitions and worries that bother us while we're awake. Drunkenness is actually a virtual recreation of that weird, often blissful state between sleep and wakefulness. Caffeine, on the other hand, is a stimulant, used for centuries to ward off drowsiness and restore alertness and concentration. It makes us feel rejuvenated, even powerful, because it wakes us up.

A chemical found in certain tropical plants, caffeine evolved as a natural insecticide, killing the bugs that fed on the plants by overstimulating their little central nervous systems. And it's very effective. At the U.S. Air Force Research Lab in Huntsville, Alabama, in 1995, scientists working for the National Aeronautics and Space Administration (NASA) recreated a well-known experiment from the 1960s in which spiders were fed various drugs to determine their effect on web building. While all of the drugs showed some effect, the spiders fed caffeine had by far the most confused and poorly constructed webs and were the most likely to die.

But humans tolerate it extremely well. While the Chinese are believed to have consumed tea in various forms for centuries, nobody really wrote down much about caffeine's effects until the fifteenth century, when (although this has been disputed) the Sufi mystic Sheikh ash-Shadhili traveled to Ethiopia and brought coffee beans back home to Yemen. He recommended them to other devout Muslims as an aid in staying awake for extended prayer sessions. It was an absolute sensation throughout the Islamic world and its enthusiasts weren't entirely limited to the most pious. It became so popular that its use was banned in Mecca in 1511 and Cairo in 1532, although both sanctions were quickly rescinded after massive public outcry.

The drink reached Europe in 1598 when Istanbul opened its first coffee house. Over the next seven decades it swept through the continent and as far away as what is now the eastern United States. As with many new crazes, coffee soon found its enemies. In 1674, the British Parliament was presented with "THE WOMEN'S PETITION AGAINST COFFEE REPRESENTING TO PUBLICK CONSIDERATION THE GRAND INCONVENIENCES ACCRUING TO THEIR SEX FROM THE EXCESSIVE USE OF THAT DRYING, ENFEEBLING LIQUOR." The anonymous pamphlet complained, among other things, that:

> The Occasion of which Insufferable Disaster, after a serious Enquiry, and Discussion of the Point by the Learned of the Faculty, we can Attribute to nothing more than the Excessive use of that Newfangled, Abominable, Heathenish Liquor called COFFEE, which Riffling Nature of her Choicest Treasures, and Drying

up the Radical Moisture, has so Eunucht our Husbands, and Crippled our more kind Gallants, that they are become as Impotent, as Age, and as unfruitful as those Desarts whence that unhappy Berry is said to be brought. For the continual sipping of this pittiful drink is enough to bewitch Men of two and twenty, and tie up the Codpice-point without a Charm. It renders them that use it as Lean as Famine, as Rivvel'd as Envy, or an old meager Hagg over-ridden by an Incubus. They come from it with nothing moist but their snotty Noses, nothing stiffe but their Joints, nor standing but their Ears.

Chronic impotence is certainly more frightening that even the mightiest hangover, still, most of us are willing to take the chance and caffeine is more popular today than ever. Not only is coffee a daily morning ritual for most people in the West, it's also now popular throughout the day and especially after meals. Caffeine also, of course, occurs in tea and many soft drinks. Some sodas even base their advertising strategy on how much caffeine their drink contains and a new category of "energy drinks" with excessive levels of the stimulant are gaining in popularity despite being linked to heart stoppages. Caffeine also occurs in low doses in chocolate, can be added to pain relievers and is now the primary active ingredient in the over-the-counter pep pills used by truckers, students and other people who need to ward off sleep artificially.

Although alcohol may have been with us longer and be more firmly embedded in our sacred and social rituals, caffeine is far more socially acceptable. While everyone will be offered coffee or tea at virtually every business meeting, see what happens if you crack open a Heineken. If you aren't fired on the spot, you'll at least be suspended. Alcohol consumption is usually limited to adults and there are parts of the world where having a stiff drink is banned, but very few refuse their children the buzz they get from a chocolate bar or a can of soda.

But it's not without risks. Expectant and nursing mothers are warned against caffeine use, as it has been linked to birth defects and other developmental problems. But most of the rest of us just drink away. I once knew a young woman who visited a doctor complaining of severe and regular headaches, aches and pains, trouble waking up and a general overall malaise. After interviewing her, he concluded that she was suffering withdrawal from long-term caffeine addiction (she had recently given up coffee). Of course, when she told us all at work, we laughed at her and told her to have a cup of coffee. Actually, her doctor was probably quite astute. Because the effects of caffeine addiction and withdrawal are so much like natural, more commonplace symptoms and few patients or doctors ever monitor caffeine intake, it usually goes undiagnosed.

While we've all felt the unpleasant effects of too much coffee, few realize that caffeine intoxication is possible and that deaths due to accidental caffeine overdoses occur regularly. According to the U.S. National Library of Medicine, too much caffeine can cause difficulty sleeping, muscle twitching, confusion, slippages in and out of consciousness, increased urination, increased thirst, fever, difficulty breathing, vomiting, diarrhea, irregular heartbeat, rapid heartbeat, hallucinations, dizziness, convulsions and even death. According to the World Health Organization, about sixty-five to seventy people die annually from caffeine toxicity or overdose, about half of them in North America. If you go to energyfiend.com, a pro-caffeine Web site and click on the "Death By Caffeine" link, you can input your weight and it will estimate how many servings of your favorite beverage will contain enough caffeine to kill you. Since my number was 304.85 cans of Diet Coke, or about 228 pounds of cola, I think I'm pretty safe.

With that reassuring news in mind, I'm still hungover and I need caffeine. Like most people in North America, I've been eating chocolate and drinking soda as long as I can remember. I had my first cup of coffee (laden with milk and sugar) at an unattended self-serve kiosk when I was nine. I've had the shakes, I've felt the bad side of caffeine and I know what it can do. But I'm always willing to take the risk.

Like a Pavolvian case study, my entire ailing body relaxes and rejoices at the hiss of the Diet Coke can opening. It's been conditioned to know that the cold, metallic smell of cola is the first step in recovery from overindulgence in alcohol the night before. As I reach for one drug to counteract the effects of another, I wonder what my grandfather did.

A giant of a man, he was a cop and later a police chief notorious for carrying a sledgehammer in the trunk of his car. He died just before I was born. I don't know as much as I'd like about him, but I do know that he drank astounding, almost historic amounts of alcohol. I think about him when I'm hungover—what it must have been like, the drinking and the stress. I think about what he must have done. No matter how much he had to drink the night before, he had to go to work the next morning and keep the peace. I don't think he reached for a Diet Coke. Maybe he took amphetamines. When he was about my age, amphetamines were legal, cheap and very popular with men who put in long hours at stressful jobs. They were often used as hangover cures by men very much like him. But I'll never know what he did. That's the problem with trying to find out about people who took amphetamines back when they were legal—they're almost all dead.

CAFFEINE ISN'T THE only chemical that plants have come up with to protect themselves. It's not the only natural stimulant used by humans, either. For thousands of years, people have been cultivating and using plants from the ephedra family. Unless you were a botanist, you probably wouldn't notice it even if you stepped on it. Generally looking like nothing more than a clump of green stems, sometimes with pairs of small green leaves or tiny flowers dotting the sides, ephedra plants grow in warm, dry climates. Enterprising people in China, India and the southwestern United States have used the plants—usually dried then prepared with water and imbibed as a tea or pounded into flour and made into tortillas—as a treatment for respiratory problems.

It was a great find.

Not only does ephedra constrict the blood vessels in the nose, thus relieving stuffiness, it also dilates the bronchial tubes, making breathing easier. For centuries, people have been drinking or otherwise consuming the ephedra plant to help them when they couldn't breathe. Native Americans who use ephedra attribute other powers to the plant, including the ability to cleanse the bloodstream, relieve backaches, heal the kidneys, settle the stomach and do at least something about pretty well any complaint people had.

But the ephedra that occurs naturally in North America is far weaker than the plant which grows in East Asia. While the members of the Cahuilla, Diegueno, Salivan, Kawaiisn and other nations that used the drug may have gotten a minor buzz, it was nothing compared to what the Chinese were enjoying. Ephedra *sinica* packed far more punch than its American cousins, ephedra *antisyphalitica* and ephedra *nevadensis*. Besides breathing easier (basically having a cure for the common cold), Asian ephedra users experienced central nervous system stimulation—an increase in energy and alertness mated with a lack of a need to sleep or eat and, if they were lucky, a feeling of increased self-esteem. The Chinese, who named the drug "ma huang," also noticed that it caused weight loss when combined with caffeine.

The drug became well established and well loved in Chinese and other Asian cultures long before it was discovered by the West and is still widely available as a traditional folk medicine.

Interestingly, one subgroup of North Americans has long been acquainted with and especially fond of native ephedrine. While the other pioneers who headed westward were fueled by regular doses of coffee and tea, the Mormons were forbidden to partake. Instead, the members of the Church of Jesus Christ of Latter-Day Saints took a page from the native people and boiled handfuls of ephedra in pots of water. They would let it steep for as long as twenty minutes and drank the broth. It was, I'm told, a sludgy, dark brown mess and is very much an acquired taste.

People began adding milk, sugar or jam to mask the natural flavor, and—dubbed "Mormon tea"—the brew became relatively popular with other pioneers, but usually only after coffee or tea supplies had run out. But it had some other positive side effects the settlers enjoyed, like relieving nasal congestion and cleansing the urinary tract.

Some also used a super-concentrated version of Mormon tea as a cure for syphilis or other venereal diseases.

Mormon tea is variously known as Brigham tea (named after Brigham Young, the charismatic Mormon who led the faithful through the American West), squaw tea, cowboy tea and, immensely more interestingly, whorehouse tea. The traditional story says that an unnamed Mormon went to a brothel called Katie's Place in Elko, Nevada, and, while he was waiting for his turn, spoke long and hard about the miraculous priapic qualities the tea provided. Before long, Katie's Place started serving the concoction, word spread and ephedra-based tea became the standard refreshment at whorehouses throughout the American West.

Amphetamine was discovered by accident. In 1887 a young Romanian scientist named Lazar Edeleanu (in many modern accounts, he's often erroneously referred to as German and his name is frequently misspelled as "Edeleano") was working on his doctoral thesis under the tutelage of Swiss chemist August Hofmann (just as often confused with Albert Hofmann, the man who invented LSD many years later) in Germany. Edeleanu isolated a compound—$C_9H_{13}N$—he called "phenylisopropylamine," but, probably because he wasn't a clinician, couldn't find any profitable applications for it. He wrote and published all the appropriate papers then promptly abandoned his discovery in search of what he thought were more lucrative pursuits.

In 1910 he discovered a cheap and efficient method of extracting sulfur dioxide from petroleum and started Edeleanu GmbH to sell his process to oil refiners. It was an immediate and huge success and the company lasted until it was bought in 2002 by Uhde, part of the immense Thyssen Krupp group of companies.

Interestingly, one of Edeleanu's students was Fritz Haber, who won the 1918 Nobel Prize in chemistry for the development of a synthetic ammonia, which could be used in fertilizers and, more potently, in explosives. Later known as "the father of chemical warfare" for his research in military poisons, Haber, a Jew, fled Germany because of Nazi persecution. Ironically, the Nazis put his life's work to use in the development of Zyklon-B, the gas used to murder their enemies, most of them Jews, in death camps like Auschwitz. He's also quite famous for inventing methylenedioxymethamphetamine, which he intended for use as a styptic—a chemical applied to a wound to stop bleeding. It wasn't until about fifty years later that somebody—actually a Manhattan-based psychoanalyst named Alexander Shulgin—decided to try swallowing it. He realized it had great powers to help people feel better and understand their problems in perspective.

Today, we call the drug "ecstasy," mostly because it makes us feel so good.

Everybody was experimenting with chemicals and after the Spanish flu epidemic of 1918–20 left at least 40 million people dead, biochemistry and pharmaceuticals became extremely lucrative businesses and no compound was left unchecked for medicinal use. One of them was amphetamine, and it turned out to be an absolute gold mine. After much experimentation, it was discovered by Smith, Kline and French (now known as GlaxoSmithKline, the second-largest pharmaceutical firm in the world) that phenylisopropylamine dilated bronchial tubes, allowing asthma, cold and allergy sufferers to breathe more easily. In 1928, the company started selling inhalers—little tubes with a cotton strip impregnated with the drug, now called amphetamine and marketed under the name Benzedrine—all over the world.

It was a huge success. One sniff of a Benzedrine inhaler could make an immense difference in one's breathing. It was one of the many wonder drugs of the era and perhaps the most impressive. There was no waiting period between dosage and effect—just snort the little tube and even the most afflicted asthmatic could breathe freely. Unfortunately, the folks at Smith, Kline and French had not put as nearly as much effort into studying the side effects of their new wonder drug as its benefits.

There were side effects.

Benzedrine users began to notice things like increased energy and stamina, a lack of a need to sleep, a decrease in appetite and an increase in sexual desire and ability.

Instead of pulling the drug off shelves, Smith, Kline and French shifted their marketing. At first, Benzedrine was prescribed to combat asthma and narcolepsy—a condition under which sufferers fall asleep involuntarily—but it was later recommended for relief of depression, Parkinson's disease, epilepsy, motion sickness, night blindness, hyperactivity, obesity, impotence and apathy. And, to make it easier to take, Benzedrine began to arrive in easy-to-swallow tablets.

Pretty soon anyone who wanted more energy or a trimmer waistline could achieve it through chemistry.

What had been side effects became selling points.

Of course, what almost nobody then (and surprisingly few people now) realized was that drugs like Benzedrine do not add chemicals to the brain, but rather just alter the flow of them. Amphetamine and other stimulants do not create or import the hormones that generate feelings of euphoria, wakefulness, power and confidence; they merely trick the brain into releasing its entire store all at once. After that, the brain must function without those hormones until more can be manufactured. The corresponding low that comes after the high can be just as intense and is usually even longer lasting. Along with the hang-overs, long-term users began to suffer from insomnia, anxiety, depression and acute psychosis.

It didn't matter; the demand for stimulants as recreational drugs skyrocketed. The United States government had declared cocaine a narcotic in 1914. The law meant cocaine would be available to most of the world only with a doctor's prescription. Other countries soon followed suit. Legions of cocaine users looked for an alternative and Benzedrine and Dexedrine (another amphetamine variant developed in the 1930s to combat hyperactivity) fit the bill. Although early amphetamines didn't quite have the kick of cocaine, the high lasted longer. More important, they were cheap, legal and widespread.

Benzedrine pills (soon known as "bennies") were not always available over the counter; so recreational amphetamine users generally used inhalers. To overcome the designed-in dosage limitations of the inhalers, users would frequently break them open to get at the Benzedrine-soaked paper or cotton strip inside. While most users would just swallow the foul-tasting contents, others would intensify the high and mask the taste by dumping the strip into a cup of coffee.

At about the same time Western pharmaceutical firms were developing amphetamine for commercial use, Japanese scientists led by Akira Ogata were developing a new compound based on Dr. Edeleanu's phenylisopropylamine. Working with Italian Francesco di Stefano in 1919, Ogata discovered a quick and easy way to synthesize a similar drug by combining ephedrine, iodine and red phosphorus. Their discovery— $C_{10}H_{15}N$—had virtually the same effects as amphetamine, but results often showed up more quickly and with much greater strength. They named it methamphetamine because it contained two quick-to-bond methyl (CH_3 or methane with a hydrogen atom removed) molecules. Quick to bond (combine with other molecules) also meant it was quick to react with human body chemistry.

During World War II, soldiers were routinely rationed "pep pills" to help combat weariness or exhaustion. When the Nazis invaded Poland to kick off the European war, they relied heavily upon speed. The soldiers of the Wehrmacht were issued pills called Pervitin. Originally introduced to the German public in 1938 as a stimulant, Pervitin was a powerful amphetamine derivative and a top seller almost as soon as it hit the market. The drug caught the attention of Otto Ranke, a military doctor and director of the Institute for General and Defense Physiology at Berlin's Academy of Military Medicine, who observed that its affects on the human psyche were very much like that of adrenalin—increasing courage, energy, self-confidence and a willingness to take risks. Perfect for an invading army, he saw it as an effective tool to help Germany win the war. In September 1939—the month Germany invaded Poland—Ranke tested the effects of Pervitin on ninety university students. The results were very encouraging.

As the Germans advanced at lightning speed across the frontier, lengthening supply lines needed to be maintained. The drug was distributed to drivers whose job it was to transport supplies and soldiers along these routes.

But success in Poland was one thing, Western Europe another. From April to June of 1940 (the period in which Germany invaded Norway, Denmark, the Netherlands, Luxembourg, Belgium and France), Berlin issued 35 million methamphetamine pills to all ranks. It worked.

But it didn't come without cost. German soldiers became addicted at epidemic rates. A look at the few letters home that remain from the era paint a disturbing picture of the state of the men in uniform. A private wrote to his parents: "It's tough out here," in November 1939, "and I hope you'll understand if I'm only able to write to you once every two to four days soon. Today I'm writing you mainly to ask for some Pervitin; Love, Hein." A couple of months later, that same soldier wrote from the heat of the invasion of France: "Perhaps you could get me some more Pervitin so that I can have a backup supply?" The same soldier, two month later, wrote to his parents: "If at all possible, please send me some more Pervitin." Private Heinrich Böll would eventually kick his Pervitin habit and turn to novel writing. In 1972 he became the first German of the post-war era to be awarded the Nobel Prize for Literature.

The salutary effect of the drug on the troops did not go unnoticed by the brass. In January 1942, in the siege of Cholm in Second Battle of Kharkov, five hundred German soldiers were surrounded by tens of thousands of Russians, temperatures that never got above 30 degrees below zero and waist-deep snow. According to the diaries of their commanding officers: "more and more soldiers were so exhausted that they were beginning to simply lie down in the snow." At that point, platoon leaders started handing out Pervitin. "After half an hour," the unit's doctor wrote in his log, "the men began spontaneously reporting that they felt better. They began marching in orderly fashion again, their spirits improved, and they became more alert." Despite overwhelming odds, the Germans escaped to fight again.

As the war wore on, it became abundantly clear that Germany didn't have the resources to fight Britain, the United States and the Soviet Union simultaneously. Well, everyone in the world knew except the Nazi hierarchy. Its demand for Pervitin escalated and desperation led to calls for an even more potent pill. On March 16, 1944, Vice-Admiral Hellmuth Heye (head of Germany's national defense committee and decades later a member of West Germany's post-war parliament) requested from central command a drug "that can keep soldiers ready for battle when they are asked to continue fighting beyond a period considered normal, while at the same time boosting their self-esteem." A noted pharmacologist from Kiel, Gerhard Orzechowski, delivered a pill he called D-IX. Along with the usual dose of three milligrams of Pervitin, it also included five milligrams of cocaine, and five milligrams of Eukodal (the military's standard and much-abused morphine-based painkiller). It arrived too late to make its way past the test stage before Germany surrendered.

That capitulation was only possible after the suicide of Germany's charismatic and fanatical leader, Adolf Hitler, a week earlier. Hitler had shown signs of mental and emotional instability early in his life. As a corporal in the German army in World War I, he was unpopular among his fellow soldiers because of his dogged obedience to their officers. Like many Germans, he believed that they were winning the war and that politicians back home (many of whom he was convinced were Marxists and/or Jews) had stabbed them in the back when they signed the Armistice ending hostilities. At about the same time news of the Armistice was hitting the front, Hitler's unit suffered a gas attack. Hitler was temporarily blinded. The doctors who treated him, however, determined that his blindness was a result not of the gas attack, but of shock—most likely the humiliating news that the Germans had surrendered. A military doctor who examined corporal Hitler called him "dangerously psychotic."

No doubt Hitler was an evil man, but there were few signs of actual mental illness until late in World War II when his closest confidantes noticed him turning into a different person. He became irritable, delusional and prone to tantrums. His body began to deteriorate rapidly and he walked only with great difficulty and his hands were constantly shaking. Maybe it was the stress, or it could have been how he chose to handle it.

IN THE 1930S, Theodor Morell was a doctor based in Dietzenbach. Although he trained in obstetrics and gynecology, he specialized in what we would now call alternative and holistic medicine. Many dismissed him as a quack, but he developed a loyal following with the wealthy and cultured, probably because of the connections he cultivated through his wife, a well-known and popular actress named Johanna Moller. He was financially well off, but as the virulently anti-semitic Nazi party rose to power, he became a target. His dark complexion and curly hair—not to mention his multiethnic clientele—led some rank-and-file Nazis to wonder if the doctor was a Jew and his practice suffered dramatically. In a cagey move designed to rescue his career, Morell managed to join the Nazi party and moved his practice to a "safer" neighborhood considered to be free of Jews.

They were smart moves that paid off right away. In the spring of 1936, Morell was visited by Heinrich Hoffmann, an intimate friend of Hitler's who was suffering from gonorrhea. Hoffmann was one of the smartest and best-connected Nazis. Hitler's favorite photographer, Hoffmann had the brilliant idea of copyrighting the Fürher's image so that both he and Hitler collected royalties every time his image was used, even on postage stamps. When Morell cured him, they became friends. In 1938, before the Nazis had overrun most of Europe, Hoffmann and his assistant Eva Braun (who would later become Hitler's wife) invited him to a party at the Berghof, Hitler's vacation home.

When Hoffman introduced Morell as his doctor, Hitler told him about a rash and some intestinal distress that his team of doctors had been unable to relieve. Sensing the import of the moment, Morell confidently told Hitler that he could cure him within the year. After seeing Morell, Hitler showed some improvement, and added the doctor to his inner circle. Others weren't as easily convinced. Hitler's second and third in command, Hermann Göring and Heinrich Himmler, considered Morell ridiculous and mocked him behind their leader's back.

Morell became part of history in 1939 when Hitler brought him along when he negotiated the annexation of the Sudetenland, a part of Czechoslovakia that many Germans had long considered part of their homeland. Hitler was determined to take the territory, but Czechoslovak president Emil Hacha was proving equally reluctant to give it up. The argument became heated. Hitler was furious. He berated Hacha with endless volleys of threat and invective. Hacha—the older of the two—reportedly became exhausted and blacked out. Morell seized the moment by injecting the unconscious Hacha with a dose of "vitamins." Within minutes, the Czechoslovak president was revived. Hitler's invective resumed, and Hacha had no choice but to surrender.

As the war dragged on and Germany's fortunes continued to decline, Morell visited Hitler more and more frequently. On each visit, the doctor gave the dictator an injection, the ingredients of which he kept secret. Hitler, in any case, grew more and more reckless, even deluded. He ordered his generals to fight to the death of the last man in hopeless situations. He commanded imaginary divisions into battle, and routinely executed anyone with the courage—or foolishness—to disagree. In the last month of the war, Morell was prescribing Hitler twenty-eight pills, two injections and a generous dose of cocaine eye drops every day. As close-range Russian artillery rained down upon his bunker, Hitler committed suicide along with his wife after shooting his dog Blondi on April 30, 1945. Germany surrendered about a week later.

After the war, Morell attempted to escape Berlin, but was captured by the Americans, who were shocked by his obesity and complete indifference to his own hygiene. Other Nazis testified that Morell had given Hitler amphetamines; he insisted to his interrogators that he'd never injected Hitler with anything but vitamins. But he was not known for his integrity and knew he probably would have been held partially responsible for Hitler's atrocities if he'd acknowledged prescribing him speed. And it's not exactly like Morell was a credible or reliable witness. As he told his wife in a letter from jail:

> As I am unable to raise my right leg or even to answer nature's call without assistance, there's probably not much they can do with me. And my head is often very muddled still and my memory has all but gone. I can't remember anything. I usually wake up around 3 or 4 a.m. and stay wide-awake until morning.

THE AMERICANS, HAVING decided Morell had exhausted his potential as a source, released the doctor in 1948. A few weeks later, the good doctor died. Did Morell prescribe Hitler amphetamines? We may never know for certain, but the specific symptoms of the Führer's mental and physical decline are tantalizing, and have convinced a number (perhaps the majority) of modern historians that he did.

FIVE OUT OF FIVE DENTISTS AGREE

While there is some debate as to why meth users lose their teeth, the American Dental Association gives its members the following information:

The oral effects of methamphetamine use can be devastating. Reports have described rampant caries [areas of progressive tooth decay] that resembles early childhood caries and is being referred to as "meth mouth". A distinctive caries pattern can often be seen on the buccal [cheekside] smooth surface of the teeth and the interproximal surfaces [where teeth touch each other] of the anterior teeth.

The rampant caries associated with methamphetamine use is attributed to the following: the acidic nature of the drug, the drug's xerostomic effect, its propensity to cause cravings for high calorie carbonated beverages, tooth grinding and clenching and its long duration of action leading to extended periods of poor oral hygiene.

Source: American Dental Association

No doubt the rise of amphetamine use after the war was driven by soldiers returning from war. But as early as 1949, medical journals were publishing articles describing instances of abuse and of addiction to the amphetamine family of drugs. Although doctors had begun to prescribe safer alternatives to amphetamines, over-the-counter use—and abuse—continued.

Benzedrine became the drug of choice for many writers from the Beat Generation like William S. Burroughs and Allen Ginsberg. Of course, they got the idea from their heroes in the jazz scene, like the legendary Charlie "Bird" Parker.

Perhaps the most noteworthy of the Beat Generation was Jack Kerouac, a former Columbia University football player who eagerly took to the drug and incorporated it into his work. As an author, Kerouac's stream-of-consciousness style seems schizophrenic to many, but his admirers compare his work to good jazz music (hence the name "Beat"). And like many jazz artists, Kerouac did his best work while high. A heavy drinker since his teen years, Kerouac was introduced to Benzedrine by Burroughs and his friend Herbert Huncke. They recommended it as a way to stay awake for prolonged writing sessions and for fighting the effects of alcohol.

After his first novel, *Town and Country*, was published to nearly complete indifference, Kerouac supposedly went on a three-week Benzedrine-fueled writing spree. The result was *On the Road*, a barely fictionalized account of his adventures while driving cross-country with his friend Neal Cassady. Using a method he called "kick writing," Kerouac fueled himself on "booze and Benzedrine" and wrote until exhausted. At one point, he typed a single 120-foot-long paragraph by continually taping another sheet of paper to the bottom of the one he'd just filled. He called it "The Roll" and it still exists. It was purchased by Indianapolis Colts owner and Kerouac fan Jim Irsay (who'd undergone his own problems with an addiction to prescription painkillers) in 2002 for $2.43 million and has since toured the United States.

But while Kerouac's feat has become well-known, less celebrated were the six years of meticulous editing the roll needed before it could be published as a novel and the terrible toll the drugs and alcohol took on his once-powerful mind and body. He died—broke, obese, angry and isolated—in the basement of his mother's Florida house in 1969. He was forty-seven and the official cause was cirrhosis of the liver.

Kerouac's legacy lived on and many creative types either dabbled in or became fully addicted to Benzedrine.

James Ellroy, the noteworthy Los Angeles-born crime writer, details his struggles with Benzedrine in his autobiography *My Dark Places*. In that period he was deluded, psychotic and blacked out frequently. He was 6-foot-3 and about 125 pounds. He was homeless for most of the time he was addicted and supported himself with shoplifting and burglary. Because he rarely ate and had few desires other than inhalers—and he'd already mastered the art of stealing them from pharmacies—the prize in many of his break-ins was nothing more than the underwear of neighborhood girls, which he would use to masturbate until he was exhausted.

"Speed heightens your sexual desire," he wrote. "You choke the chicken for twelve hours at a pop—it almost killed me."

Only the deprivation provided by a jail term that coincided with a severe bout of pneumonia set Ellroy on the road to recovery.

MORE RECENT HISTORY: BENZEDRINE GOES HOLLYWOOD

THE FRENCH HAD PROVED unable to hold onto their colonies in what they called Indo-China, so by the Fifties the Americans stepped in in an attempt to prop up the unstable pro-Western governments that had taken hold in South Vietnam, Laos and Cambodia. It started slowly at first as President John F. Kennedy sent military advisors to the countries to help train their fledgling armed forces.

Kennedy had been a hero in World War II, rescuing three shipmates after their patrol boat had been rammed by a Japanese destroyer. But the feats of that night severely aggravated the problems Kennedy already had with his back. Actually, despite the youthful vigor he portrayed as president, Kennedy had numerous health problems, including an adrenal problem called Addison's disease and a gastrointestinal ailment called celiac disease. As a child, he suffered from scarlet fever, diphtheria and whooping cough, and had acid reflux, allergies and knee problems as an adult. He was so chronically ill, in fact, that he was hospitalized on more than three dozen occasions and given

the last rites three times. During the 1960 presidential campaign, advisor Ted Sorenson noted that his hands trembled and
that he seemed "tired" and not "clear." After he won the election,
Kennedy is reputed to have fallen asleep while interviewing a
candidate for secretary of agriculture.

Kennedy is said to have combated his health problems with
massive doses of steroids and other drugs. While it hasn't been
proven, there is strong evidence that Kennedy was also a frequent user of amphetamines. He was, according to many, a
patient of Max Jacobson, a physician who later became famous
as "Dr. Feelgood" for his habit of prescribing and injecting many
noted Hollywood celebrities with speed. Jacobson even visited
the president during the peak of the Cuban Missile Crisis.

Many historians now also believe that Kennedy was high on
speed when he gave the defiant speech in West Berlin in which
he stated "Ich bein ein Berliner" and rallied the West against
Soviet incursion. A recent article in *The Atlantic* said that when
the president was asked about Jacobson's injections, he said: "I
don't care if it's horse piss; it works." Not everybody agreed.
"Looking back on it, it's amazing how we all just accepted the
fact that the president was taking Dr. Feelgood with him to a
meeting that would affect the entire world," wrote singer Eddie
Fisher, a good friend of the president's, in his autobiography.
"The fate of the free world rested on Max's injections. I can still
see Max taking a little from this bottle, a little from that one, and
pull down your pants, Mr. President."

As details of the president's drug use made their way to the
public in the years after his assassination, the mainstream
media took a finger-wagging tone. A 1972 article in *The New
York Times* quoted one of Kennedy's doctors as disapproving of
the president's amphetamine use and saying: "No president
with his finger on the red button has any business taking stuff
like that."

He wasn't the only Western head of state taking speed. Anthony Eden, Winston Churchill's successor as prime minister of Great Britain, is said by noted historian Hugh Thomas to have "lived on Benzedrine." After a botched gallbladder operation damaged his bile duct, Eden was prescribed Benzedrine, which was a commonly used restorative at the time. When Egyptian forces under the command of charismatic strongman Gamal Abdel Nasser took control of the Suez Canal in 1956, threatening Europe's supply of petroleum imports, British, French and Israeli forces stepped in. While the military action was successful, the U.S. (dedicated to a philosophy of decolonialism), Canada and other countries pressured the Europeans to withdraw. Eden enraged international opinion and actually managed to create a bizarre situation in which both the U.S. and U.S.S.R. were aligned against him and his allies. Making matters worse, he shocked the world by going on what his government called "a vacation." After the Soviets threatened to fire a massive salvo of missiles (they weren't specific about whether they would be nuclear-armed or not) at London if British forces didn't withdraw immediately, U.S. president Dwight Eisenhower got Eden on the phone and managed to get him to pull back his troops without even consulting his French and Israeli allies. Eden's biographers now generally agree that he went to Jamaica to kick the Benzedrine habit that was seriously affecting his health and already unstable emotional state. He resigned from office soon after returning to Britain. The Suez Crisis marked the last time Britain exerted its strategic will without U.S. assistance (unless you count the 1982 Falklands War, which had the tacit approval of the Americans) and the end of the era in which individual European countries were considered serious players in geopolitics.

Kennedy may have been using amphetamines to battle health problems. But it was a different story for the thousands of soldiers being shipped off to Vietnam. It was a grueling, non-stop twenty-four-hour guerilla war. To keep up, or maybe simply to relieve the pressure and strain, soldiers on both sides turned to various types of speed, including *ma huang*, amphetamines and methamphetamines.

Thousands of soldiers returning home returned as addicts.

American veterans of Vietnam returned to a society, however, that had become largely intolerant of amphetamines. After stories of abuse became commonplace, the U.S. Food and Drug Administration outlawed over-the-counter sales of amphetamine-based stimulants. It was (and is) still available by prescription, but the days of Benzedrine parties at the coffee shop were over.

But other events in the last half of the twentieth century also led to the continued, if not increased, abuse of amphetamines. Many of the cities and especially the ports of Southeast Asia had been occupied by the Japanese in World War ii. Those that hadn't been exposed to stimulants before the war soon were. When the war ended, the Japanese military had warehouses full of meth pills but no soldiers who needed them. The stocks were released to the general public and caused an epidemic. It got so bad, in fact, that the World Health Organization estimated that there were more than two million speed addicts in Japan in the 1950s before the government got serious about controlling the drug. Although use has declined significantly since then, the drug (locally called "shabu" is still popular among truck drivers, college students and teenage girls who are trying to lose weight) is still a major problem. Not only is addiction commonplace— the United Nations Office on Drugs and Crime (unodc) reported in 2005 that Japan is "one of the most lucrative markets" for meth—but trade in shabu has led to the financing and continued success of the Yakuza, the crime organization that controls trade in the drug.

Most of the Asian countries that had been exposed to speed by the Japanese had little or no access to large pharmaceutical factories, local users became freelance chemists, transforming whatever they had into amphetamines. As the war escalated, they shared their recipes and techniques with the Americans, who brought them home.

Using standard scientific equipment and commonplace ingredients, clandestine speed makers found that they could not only supply their own needs, but make a few bucks as well. But it was a small-time business—basically friends supplying friends—until 1965.

Shortly after World War II, a few combat veterans settled in California and isolated themselves from the general population. They wore leather jackets, rode Harley-Davidsons, drank lots of beer, threw wild parties and beat the crap out of anyone who got in their way. While they ultimately faded away, they inspired many disaffected young men to emulate their style and way of life. Before long, legions of young men started wearing leather jackets, affecting an alienated attitude and riding motorcycles. The most notorious, with chapters in San Bernardino and Oakland, California, called themselves the Hells Angels.

Something about the name, the death's head emblem and the charisma of their leadership set the Hells Angels apart from the hundreds of other motorcycle gangs in California. While the strict leadership of the gang frowned upon the use and sale of illegal drugs, many Hells Angels supplemented their incomes with small-time drug sales, dealing mostly in locally or Mexican-grown marijuana. But things changed in 1965. After the club's annual "run" in Monterey, two teenage girls claimed to have been gang-raped by members of the Hells Angels. Four prominent and easily identified members were arrested. Facing huge legal fees, the club's leadership needed to raise cash. According to sources within the club, one courageous member spoke highly of a friend of his who had made tons of money making and selling speed.

The club's leadership, the source suggested, at first was against it. They had investigated the suggestion before, but didn't like the fact that their supply of drugs would be dependent on foreign suppliers. There were too many "ifs" involved.

Amphetamines were different.

Here was a drug that could be easily manufactured using materials purchased from a pharmacy or hardware store. There were no foreigners or foreign cartels involved. After much deliberation, the Hells Angels decided to go into the speed business.

It was an immediate success. Despite some initial reluctance, the jingoistic and homophobic bikers even found ready and willing customers in the growing antiwar and gay movements. The once-impoverished Hells Angels were now wealthy and envied throughout the biker world. Soon Hells Angels chapters began springing up all over the U.S., Canada, the U.K., Australia and Scandinavia and pretty well all of them have been linked to the distribution of illegal stimulants. As the reach of the bikers expanded, so did the demand for speed. Rival gangs, such as the Outlaws in Chicago, the Pagans in Baltimore, the Bandidos in Houston and the Mongols in Los Angeles copied the Hells Angels' look, culture and ability to make money by selling drugs. While the other gangs weren't as reluctant to sell imported drugs, they all depended on amphetamines—and later crystal meth—as their big moneymaker. As the demand for amphetamines grew, driving retail prices higher, experienced "cooks" became exceedingly valuable and were actively sought, diligently recruited and often handsomely rewarded by bikers interested in making quick money.

While it was originally hippies, gay men, entertainers and other counterculture types who sought the drug, the bikers eventually found many new places to sell amphetamines. At the time, much of Southern California's population consisted of poor, blue-collar whites who had migrated from other parts of the country in search of agricultural or factory jobs during the Depression. Much like the Joad family in John Steinbeck's *The Grapes of Wrath*, millions of displaced families emerged from what were basically refugee camps into what became the towns and cities surrounding Los Angeles. But right from the beginning, these new migrants encountered resistance and discrimination from the locals. Easily identified by their accents and their poverty, refugees from the Prairies were called "Okies," while those who came from the Deep South were known as "Rednecks" and "Peckerwoods." Not only did they have a hard time getting anything but the most menial and lowest-paying jobs, but California even passed an "anti-Okie" law in 1937, which allowed the police to jail any indigent person who could not prove state residency.

Although the law was repealed in 1941 and many migrant families found prosperity during and after World War II, the descendants of the Okies and other poor whites didn't forget the cold welcome they received from the locals, the government and especially the police, who could be—and often were—quite brutal. A culture developed not exactly of lawlessness, but of mistrusting the establishment and subverting it whenever they could. Many familiar countercultural archetypes—the greaser, the beatnik, the biker especially—originated with this group.

There were other factors that joined in the confluence that made speed a prominent, if not the dominant, drug among Californians at that time. Just as amphetamines were establishing a foothold in the continental U.S. (it had been become established in Asian-identified Hawaii much earlier), authorities were cracking down on the importation and distribution of cocaine, a drug they considered far more dangerous. Major busts and seizures reduced the amount of coke available and pushed its retail price way up. Those who could find it often couldn't afford it and turned to speed as a cheaper, easier-to-get alternative.

While coke users were turning to amphetamines in huge numbers, so were heroin addicts. Increasingly through the middle part of the 1960s, doctors would use amphetamine derivatives to treat narcotic users. While speed no doubt eased the symptoms of heroin withdrawal and allowed many addicts to affect a look of normalcy, if not exactly health, the end result in many cases was that the doctors relieved one addiction, but supplanted it with another.

One of the most famous users was comedian Lenny Bruce. Show business mythology has it that Bruce tired of buying speed on the street and used his abundant charm to convince a besotted gay doctor into writing him both a prescription for injectable amphetamines and a letter explaining his possession of drugs or syringes. It didn't help. In 1961, Bruce was arrested for possession of amphetamines in Philadelphia, but served no jail time. He was arrested for speed a second time. Bruce acted as his own attorney and was convicted and sentenced to a year in prison. While out on bail, his lawyers managed to overturn the decision. But by this time Bruce's addiction was taking its heavy toll. His act turned less funny and more bitter and offensive. His trademark caustic wit and brilliant commentary degenerated into wandering, tedious and even paranoid attacks on anyone he thought had wronged him.

On August 3, 1966, he died. He was sitting on a toilet in his Hollywood Hills home, naked except for a silk sash tied around his arm. There were syringes on the floor and the police who investigated the scene told the press he died of an overdose of "a narcotic, probably heroin." When the medical examiner stated the next day that the cause of death was unknown and their tests for drugs inconclusive, Bruce's fans speculated that he died of other causes or was killed by police. Bruce's friend Phil Spector—an eccentric record producer who was later said to have pointed loaded firearms at John Lennon, Leonard Cohen and Joey Ramone—said the actual cause of Bruce's death was "an overdose of police." (In 2003 the sixty-two-year-old Spector was arrested for the murder of actress Lana Clarkson. When faced with life in prison, he said he shot her because of his own drug problems.)

Speed—which increased energy, self-esteem and libido—mated perfectly with the "swinging" ethos of white suburban California. They worked hard all day and came home dedicated to party. And it was cool. At first. Most celebrities who used amphetamines (like the Beatles, Johnny Cash and Elvis Presley) did their best to keep their habits secret, but many people who knew them or worked with them were aware of drug use—even fictional characters were free to use it as often as they liked.

Perhaps the most profoundly admired character of the era was British superspy/ladies' man James Bond. A creation of author Ian Fleming, Bond appealed to a broad range of readers and moviegoers because of his roguish attitude and his polished, flawless charm, commanding intellect and devastating, sexually-charged wit to escape dangerous situations and to seduce exotic and beautiful women. While he generally expressed a fondness for martinis (giving rise to his famous if seemingly backward tagline "shaken, not stirred"), he was not above taking speed. Amphetamines are mentioned in a positive context in three different James Bond books and are featured almost as a secret weapon in *Moonraker*:

> "Benzedrine," said James Bond. "It's what I shall need
> if I'm going to keep my wits about me tonight. It's apt
> to make one a bit overconfident, but that'll help too." He
> stirred the champagne so that the white powder whirled
> among the bubbles. Then he drank the mixture down

with one long swallow. "It doesn't taste," said Bond, "and the champagne is quite excellent."

In southern California neighborhoods at the time, "getting some" was often as easy as slipping a few bucks to the next-door neighbor, the milkman or the guy who fixed your car. But these were mere middlemen making a quick buck. Cooking amphetamine was just too dangerous for most suburbanites. By the middle sixites the "cool" had lost its flavor: speed use had become so identified with truckers, bikers and white trash that it was eschewed by the jet-set and hip wannabes.

The first speed lab busted by police in California was in Santa Cruz, which in 1967 was a sleepy town south of San Francisco. According to Larry, a retired bookstore owner who used to, as he says, "help out" at the Haight-Ashbury Free Clinic in San Francisco, the clinic's staff—mostly hippies—took an uncharacteristically intolerant stance to speed.

"It didn't really mesh with what we were about then," Larry told me. "Speed freaks were all about themselves and getting more, more, more...it was disturbing, really, kind of militaristic." Later in our conversation, throughout which he smoked pot and digressed into endless tangents, he admitted that he thought that only "white trash" ever used speed.

The white trash image took hold. Police departments and prisons in California began to associate tattooed meth users and cooks with white supremacist groups. This further helped establish the stereotype of the meth addict as white, rural and mostly covered in tattoos.

In a landmark speech in 1971, U.S. president Richard Nixon called illegal drug use "public enemy number one," and two years later Congress created the Drug Enforcement Agency (DEA) as a separate and powerful entity within the Department of Justice. Their mandate was to organize police throughout the

country in a nationwide crackdown on drug possession, manufacture and importation. Because speed had only been made
illegal to sell over the counter for a decade, it may have been considered by law enforcement as less serious a threat than its more
familiar cousins, marijuana, cocaine, heroin and LSD. In an
effort to dissuade people from the idea that amphetamines were
a safe alternative to other drugs, the DEA did come up with the
snappy slogan "speed kills." Most people now associate the
phrase more with highway speed than the drug.

For decades, amphetamine derivatives remained the drug of
choice for a very small section of the population. But like so
many other cultural phenomena that emerged in California at
the time—like fast food and motorcycle gangs—speed use gradually expanded eastward. The primary vectors were biker gangs
and truck drivers, who often used it to stay alert for long hauls.
Most amphetamines were still consumed by the same kind of
poor, non-urban white people who made them.

In fact, as the culture turned towards personal fulfillment
and free expression in the seventies (often called "the me
decade") and the "go-go" eighties, a new drug entered the scene.
People yearned for the respect and even envy of their neighbors
and peers. Who wanted to be associated with a drug that con-
jured up images of bikers, truckers and rednecks?

Many of the successful businessmen, performers and urban
gay men who had previously been a small but lucrative market
for speed switched to cocaine.

Seductive in part because it was imported, popular with the
jet set in Europe and expensive, influential people started using
cocaine in huge amounts and fans who wanted to be like them
followed suit. Although speed retained its popularity among its
core crowd—the lower middle-class whites in small towns in
southern and western United States—it was totally eclipsed by
cocaine everywhere else.

One notable exception was the brilliant mathematician Paul Erdös. Born Erdös Pál in Hungary in 1913, he was quickly recognized as a child prodigy when—at four years old—he started performing feats like correctly calculating the number of seconds his parents and friends had been alive. The rising tide of anti-Semitism in Eastern Europe drove him first to England in 1934, then to the U.S. in 1938, where he accepted a professorship at Princeton University, the same school that employed Albert Einstein.

Long considered an eccentric, Erdös drank remarkable amounts of coffee and his thin, continually trembling body housed a magnificent mind that became increasingly hard for others to follow. Things peaked in 1971 when, in an effort to alleviate some of the grief he felt over the death of his beloved mother, he turned to amphetamines. Although he continued to produce brilliant and elegant theorems, his behavior became increasingly odd. Erdös developed his own vocabulary and often refused to work with those who hadn't learned it. He developed a hatred of God, whom he called the Supreme Fascist, because Erdös believed there was a heavenly book of divine mathematical theorems God was petulantly keeping away from him. He also accused God of hiding his socks and important papers.

His friends and peers became concerned. Ron Graham, Erdös' best friend and an extraordinary mathematician in his own right, was taking care of the professor's finances when he noticed the large sums he was spending on amphetamines, which he was by the late 1970s taking every day. Convinced that some time away from the drug would clear his friend of his addiction, Graham offered the highly competitive Erdös $500 if he could stay off speed for a month. Erdös managed it, but hated it, complaining that it put his work back a month. "Before, when I looked at a blank piece of paper my mind was filled with ideas," he said. "Now all I see is a blank piece of paper."

Although Erdös never stopped using amphetamines until his death in 1996, he didn't advocate them for others. When a profile of him was published in the November 1987 issue of *The Atlantic*, Erdös called the author and scolded him.

"You shouldn't have mentioned the stuff about Benzedrine," he said. "It's not that you got it wrong. It's just that I don't want kids who are thinking about going into mathematics to think you have to take drugs to succeed."

Other drugs were coming onto the market as well.

"In addition to the cocaine coming in from Colombia, we were beginning to see a lot of large seizures, a ton or more, of something called Quaalude pills," said Gene Haislip, deputy assistant administrator of the DEA, referring to much-publicized cocaine seizures in the early 1980s. "I really wasn't familiar with that drug, so I called technical experts, and I said, 'What the hell is this, and what's going on?'"

Developed by Indian researcher M.L. Gujiral during the malaria crisis of 1955, methaqualone was later marketed in the West as a sleeping pill under a variety of names, including Quaalude. The name is said to have derived from the phrase "quiet interlude," which the marketing team at William H Rohrer, Inc. believed had a soothing quality. The double "a" was inserted because the same company had so much success with another product, an antacid named Maalox.

Because Quaaludes gave users a feeling of euphoria along with its relaxing qualities, it quickly became a popular recreational drug. But it was habit-forming. Overdoses resulting in coma and death from cardiac arrest became frequent enough that it was named a Schedule II Controlled Substance in the U.S. in 1973, meaning that it would henceforth be available only by prescription and that all manufacture, importation and sale would be monitored by the agency. After plunging in popularity for about a decade, Quaaludes were reintroduced to the market by Colombian cartels who needed a lower-cost alternative to cocaine and one that didn't need to be shipped in bulky quantities like marijuana. It very quickly became popular with high schoolers, and even led to a popular song by Shel Silverstein, called "Quaaludes Again," about a girl who "fumbles and stumbles and falls down the stairs / makes love to the leg of the dining room chair."

But Quaaludes were very low on the DEA's list of priorities until Haislip started making noise about it. He asked his staff how much they estimated was being consumed in the U.S.

"They said, 'Well, about seven tons a year.' I said: 'Well, how the hell can that be? We've already seized seven tons in the last three or four weeks.'"

He immediately went to work. Through investigation, he found that the illegal Quaaludes on the street were not made in the U.S., but were actually manufactured in Colombia and modeled to look like commonplace prescription sleeping pills. He also quickly discovered that facilities to make methaqualone did not exist in Colombia, so he correctly surmised that there must be large quantities of the active ingredient being imported from other countries. He went to Colombia and, after much investigation, was able to make a seizure of a shipment of Quaaludes being loaded from a dock in Baranquilla. Luckily, he also found paperwork that linked the methaqualone to a factory in Hungary.

Haislip put together all the evidence he could—"photographs, copies of paperwork, everything we needed, a complete analysis of the problem"—and flew to Hungary. Much to his surprise, the Hungarian authorities he met with not only acknowledged that their methaqualone was being used to manufacture illegal Quaaludes, but also agreed that it was immoral and reprehensible. The Hungarians not only promised to stop the export of the chemical, they actually called back a shipment that was already in Switzerland on its way to South America. "As far as they were concerned, there would be no further problem from Hungary with regard to that drug," Haislip said. "This was an amazing achievement to me."

Armed with this knowledge and encouraged by his early success, Haislip tracked down every factory in the world that was sending the Colombians methaqualone and showed them his evidence. Of course, not every factory and not every country was as willing to deal with the DEA as the Hungarians were, but within a few years, Haislip and his team had binding agreements with factories in Austria, West Germany and even the People's Republic of China to keep the chemical out of the cartels' hands.

With no methaqualone, the cooks in Colombia had no way to make Quaaludes. Almost overnight, a $2 billion-per-year industry evaporated into nothing.

"At one time it was as big as the heroin or cocaine problem, and people wonder why it's gone away," Haislip said. "It's gone away because we beat them." Although opponents of the War on Drugs may attribute the virtual extinction of illegal Quaaludes to other factors, it would appear that Haislip's efforts and the eradication were not merely coincidental. They do, however, have a point when it comes to the commonly held opinion that the dearth of Quaaludes may have sent users looking for other, potentially more dangerous drugs.

Despite the fact that far more attention was being paid to more glamorous drugs, the DEA made its first real attempt at managing the speed problem in the United States in 1980, three years before Haislip attacked Quaaludes. The publication of an amphetamine recipe book called *The Whole Drug Manufacturer's Catalog* (by an author with the delightfully juvenile pseudonym of Chewbacca Darth) came to the attention of the agency, and revealed that most clandestine labs used phenyl-2-propanone as the primary active ingredient in the manufacture of amphetamines. Also known as phenylacetone, phenyl-2-propanone is an organic compound, usually a clear yellowish liquid, which is used for various applications, from the manufacture of medicine to the recipe for some rat poisons. On February 11, 1980, the DEA managed to have phenyl-2-propanone declared a Schedule 11 Controlled Substance.

The plan backfired in a colossal fashion. Deprived of their phenyl-2-propanone, speed cooks reverted to Plan B. The Japanese had cooked their speed with ephedrine. Not only did it work, it was a panacea. The new product, called methamphetamine or simply "meth," had at least double the potency of the old stuff and was cheaper and easier to produce.

"From a chemical perspective, methamphetamine is amphetamine with a methyl group, if you're interested in the science of it," said Rob Bovett, legal counsel for the Oregon Narcotics Enforcement Association. "But it's pretty much like a high-octane gasoline versus a low-octane gasoline—methamphetamine, of course, is the high-octane version." He's understating the case. Pretty well everyone I've talked to about comparing the new drug has struggled to find an appropriate metaphor to indicate how much more powerful the new drug was. One person who has tried both drugs told me that "if amphetamine was like a sixty-watt bulb, meth is like Las Vegas." And, as though that wasn't enough, the ephedrine in the recipe could be replaced with cheaper, even easier-to-acquire pseudoephedrine (the active ingredient in most over-the-counter cold remedies) with no loss in potency or volume.

The discovery of the ephedrine and pseudoephedrine method led to a bizarre urban myth. The emergence of factory poultry farms after World War 11 yielded greater numbers of birds with far more usable meat than had ever been available before, and retail prices dropped accordingly. From 1950 to 1970 chicken meat consumption more than doubled in the U.S. and Canada and increased as much as fivefold in countries like Australia. According to the urban legend, farmers had laced the chicken feed with ephedrine. Enterprising speed cooks, the rumors continued, would steal the pure ephedrine from chicken farms. The problem is, commercial chicken feed has never contained stimulants. In 1990, Dr. Roger A. Ely wrote a report for *The Journal of Forensic Science* in which he detailed the fact that no evidence existed that feed producers had ever added stimulants to their product. In fact, in quite the reverse, the Albers Feed Company (now known as Manna Pro Corporation), actually added *sedatives* to its meal in order to help chickens cope with the hysteria associated with the confines and confusion of factory farming. Still, the myth of stimulated chickens persists and there are many mentions of cooks using "chicken speed" and even published accounts of cooks who have stolen "fifty-pound drums of pure ephedra and shotguns" from chicken farms. Perhaps even more amusing is the fact that, in his research, Ely came across a significant number of misinformed souls who had approached feed company personnel in search of often ridiculously huge quantities of ephedra to "feed to their chickens."

Still, the relative abundance and cheapness of ephedrine and pseudoephedrine is a primary factor that led to the ascendancy of meth. Meth is small and easy to conceal. It came in two distinct forms depending on whether it was in crystal form or powder. Originally, the solid was called "crystal meth" and the powder "crank," but the terms are now largely considered interchangeable and just two of many pseudonyms. The term "crank" is said by many to derive from a practice bikers had of hiding it in the crankcases of their Harleys. Considering how simple it is to hide even large doses of meth in other spots and how full of oil crankcases are and how messy and complicated they are to get into, it would seem that the name actually came from the way the drug "cranks" up its users.

The crystalline form resembled small shards of glass, mica or rock candy. Generally a dirty white color, although it could be colored by impurities, the chunks were translucent and generally varied in size from very tiny to as big as a fingernail.

The less pure, usually white, powdered form was also available. It was usually ingested by swallowing—capsules designed for other pills that would be emptied and filled with meth—or mixed into a beverage. The resulting brew was often called "biker coffee." More serious users could snort it like cocaine, smoke it in a pipe or inject it into their veins.

Fresh from his success with Quaaludes, Haislip and his team took on meth. It seemed to him like a pretty easy job...at first. After all, the key ingredients were ephedrine or pseudoephedrine and the world's supply came from just nine factories in what were basically friendly countries, and there were nowhere near as many Americans who used meth as had used Quaaludes.

"We had extremely good reception on the part of this proposal, both from the president, the Justice Department and the Congress," said Haislip. "However, it did soon surface that legitimate industry had concerns."

NOTHING SUCCEEDS
LIKE EXCESS:
THE CARTELS

IT TURNS OUT THAT those "legitimate concerns"
centered around the huge and entirely legal use of pseudoephedrine and, to a lesser extent, ephedrine. Lobbyists from
the pharmaceutical industry shifted into overdrive and appeared
to change the government's mind. The bill began to meet with
a great deal of opposition. Haislip was clearly disappointed, but
philosophical. "They live in the business community, where the
name of the game is to make money and sell product, supposedly for legitimate purposes, whereas we in law enforcement,
we see the other side of it," he said. "We see the harm that these
same drugs and chemicals can do when they slip from the legitimate to the illicit."

The arguments between the DEA and the pharmaceutical
industry went on for years. Finally, in 1989, they hammered out
a deal—all pseudoephedrine and ephedrine imported into the
country would have to be reported to the DEA, but no retail sales
of drugs containing the chemicals would be. The negotiations
continued to be acrimonious.

"We felt the DEA was confused about who was the bad guy," said Allan Rexinger, a lobbyist for the pharmaceutical industry and a key part of the team that created the bill. "It was our feeling that what they were really saying to us was: 'We're from the DEA, and this is the way it's got to be, and if over-the-counter medicines have to go down the tubes, well, that's just too bad.'"

Haislip and the DEA were determined to curb the meth problem before it exploded. "I remember being at one of the meetings with industry, and a representative of one of the well-known chemical houses, he stood up and he said: 'Mr. Haislip, you don't understand. That's not the way we do business. We get orders over the telephone. We don't know who's at the other end.' I said: 'No, you don't understand. That's not the way you're doing business anymore.'"

The effect was immediate and profound. Ephedrine powder, which had been ridiculously cheap before the legislation, started selling on the street for almost as much as cocaine. "They were desperate," said Haislip.

But the DEA often measures its success in other ways. Haislip and his crew diligently scanned arrest, hospitalization and death rates for people who might have used speed from 1990 to 1992. They were encouraged to see how quickly and how far the rates had dropped.

But things changed.

Cocaine, once considered the drug of choice for the rich and famous, by this time had fallen on hard times. In fact, it was a victim of its own success. In an effort to make even more money off the coca leaf, cooks had started to mix cocaine with ammonia. After evaporating the excess moisture, the cocaine was transformed into a rock-like substance, which was cheap and could be smoked for an intense, if brief, high. When lit, the new substance produced a distinct cracking noise, leading to the name "crack." Not surprisingly, it proved very popular.

Suddenly, cocaine was in the hands of anyone who could find a five dollar bill.

Few, however, were prepared for how addictive it could be. Before too long, most American cities were overrun with a new breed of cocaine addicts. Previously, the drug had been associated with the rich, famous and successful; now it showed itself in the person of the "crackhead"—a poor, unemployed and often homeless person who made it clear that they were willing to do anything, no matter how degrading or illegal, for another hit. Crime, especially petty stuff like holdups and random thefts, skyrocketed. Crackheads were stealing everything that wasn't nailed down and prying up plenty of what was. And the people who sold them crack were shooting it out in the streets to deter-

---

WHO'S TAKING METH?

In an effort to make sentencing more fair, the U.S. Sentencing Commission, part of the Department of Justice, studied the demographic statistics of meth arrests. The study was made in 1998, but later surveys indicate similar results:

"Overall, more than 80 percent of the offenders are male and nearly three-quarters are United States citizens. Among Hispanic offenders however, only 28.0 percent are citizens. The race/ethnicity of these offenders differs somewhat by the form of the drug used at sentencing. Generally, African Americans represent a very small proportion of these offenders, regardless of form, and the bulk of methamphetamine offenders are white or of Hispanic origin. If the form of the drug is Ice [crystal meth], Asians account for nearly two-thirds (62.7 percent) of these cases. However, Asians account for very few cases among the other forms of the drug. When the form of the drug is methamphetamine-mix, the majority of cases are white (69.2 percent) followed at some distance by Hispanics (27.4 percent). When the form is methamphetamine-actual the proportion of whites and Hispanics is equal (47.4 percent white; 47.2 percent Hispanic)."

Source: United States Sentencing Commission

mine who had the right to sell the incredibly lucrative drug where. Before too long, terms like "crack baby" and "crack whore" became arguably the worst insults in the American vernacular. In a few years, cocaine went from awesome to awful. Demand for cocaine plunged.

Not all of the illegal drug manufacturers and distributors were entirely disappointed by cocaine's fall from grace. One of the second-echelon cocaine cartels, Mexico's Amezcua Brothers, saw an opportunity. For years, the brothers—Luis Amezcua-Contreras and Jose de Jesus Amezcua-Contreras, who everyone called "Jesus"—had long been middlemen for the Colombian cocaine cartels. The brothers first made a name for themselves (they were originally known as "the Colima Gang") by smuggling immigrants into the United States. After a while they began to realize they could make much more money if those immigrants carried marijuana over the border with them. That business quickly evolved into cocaine smuggling, as the powder was much easier to conceal and produced much higher profits. The Amezcuas started to buy large amounts of cocaine from the Colombians, then import it to the U.S. on the backs of immigrants to be sold by connections, mostly Mexican citizens, there. The Colombians bought old passenger planes, typically Boeing 727s, gutted them, packed them full of cocaine and sent them to Guadalajara. They would return stuffed with millions of dollars in cash. The Mexicans, on the other hand, had a significantly more dangerous job, with well-equipped and heavily armed DEA agents patrolling the border, Although the profit margins were ridiculously high compared to legitimate businesses, they were nothing like the obscene profits the Colombians were making. And, the Amezcuas also had to pay huge amounts of their own cash (or drugs) to Mexican police, customs officials, judges, prosecutors and politicians to turn a blind eye to the daily flights back and forth to Colombia, which had no passengers and no official cargo.

The secret to making the big money, the brothers came to realize, was *making* the drugs, not retailing.

Unfortunately, the Mexican climate was not suitable for coca leaves, the key ingredient in cocaine, and the Colombians controlled pretty much everywhere it could grow. Cocaine was out; they needed an alternative. They dealt a little marijuana, which grew well in Mexico, but also grew well in California. That market was saturated. Besides, it took tons of weed to make the same amount of cash a pound or so of cocaine would yield.

With ephedrine imports to the United States now closely monitored, American speed users were going hungry. And a new generation of potential drug users were too scared by what they had seen crack do to ever try cocaine. After much thought and deliberation, the Guadalajara-based Amezcuas correctly guessed that the market for speed was huge and largely untapped. And, since imports of ephedrine to Mexico were barely examined, let alone controlled, the potential to corner the market hung tantalizingly within reach.

The brothers began acquiring huge quantities of the chemical—all of it legitimately—from factories in Germany, India, the Czech Republic and Switzerland. At first, they resold the ephedrine to established cooks and business was brisk, but the Amezcuas tired of sharing profits again. Their solution was ingenious. The brothers began to import not just ephedrine, but cooks as well. Trained in Mexico using recipes taken from books like Darth's, the cooks perfected the manufacture of meth before sending it north. Before long, the Amezcuas had established huge meth facilities throughout California. They chose to make the drugs in California simply because the penalty for importing ephedrine into the U.S. was a misdemeanor but importing meth was a felony.

"We went from a meth problem in California controlled primarily by specific groups like outlaw bikers to seeing industrial-sized factories set up in California," said Robert Pennal, head of the Meth Task Force for the Fresno Police Department. "We started seeing it out in our deserts; we started seeing it all throughout the Central Valley, where these organizations fit in well with the farm labor community."

And they had an astute organization plan as well. According to investigators, Luis and Jesus rarely traveled outside Mexico and never on business. They surrounded themselves with family—mostly cousins and in-laws—who they knew would never turn informant and would definitely take the fall for them if things got ugly. That circle of managers gave orders to another level of family and close friends who told the actual workers—the importers, exporters, cooks and distributors—what to do. The people who actually came in contact with the drugs and raw material, those who constantly risked prosecution, were often so far removed from the inner workings that they had no idea who their employers were. If they were caught, they could only inform on the level above them. And even that was exceptionally rare, because it carried the threat of extremely dire consequences.

"Cheap and sometimes coerced Mexican labor from across the border was imported into California to run large-scale commercial laboratory operations under the direction of several key personnel," said Katina Kypridakes, Criminal Intelligence Specialist Supervisor for the California Department of Justice Bureau of Narcotic Enforcement.

The brothers were also astute enough to ensure that their managers maintained a workforce free of meth users—they just couldn't be trusted.

"They had established family networks there," Pennal said. "These are individuals that weren't meth users—these were people who were in it strictly for the business."

And business was booming. Because of the standardization provided by their network of factories and organized manufacturing methods and the pharmaceutical-quality ephedrine they imported, the meth that the Amezcuas produced was far more powerful than had been seen on the street before. According to the Rand Corporation, a Santa Monica-based thinktank, the purity of street-level meth doubled from 1991 to 1994, reaching a frighteningly potent 70 percent.

Demand, much of it coming from crack and cocaine users, rose to meet production, and it was huge. While the cooks in the "redneck" labs measured their output in ounces, the "superlabs" (as the police called them) generally dealt in units of at least one hundred pounds.

"The Amezcua brothers revolutionized the meth trade—they turned it from a small mom-and-pop backyard operation to an industrial-scale production line," said Steve Suo, an award-winning investigative reporter for *The Oregonian* who has written extensively about meth. "They made possible the super-lab, which is capable of producing 1,500 times what an ordinary user can make for himself." They were so successful and inno-vative that their achievement has often, usually grudgingly, been compared to how Henry Ford established a workable auto industry. The authorities use various statistics to determine how popular a drug is becoming. According to California Democratic senator Dianne Feinstein, "Meth-related emergency room admissions increased 269 percent from 1992 to 1994." Similarly, the rates of people entering rehab and arrested for meth-related offenses grew at about the same proportion.

That efficiency also translated to distribution. In a large part because most speed cooks were, to put it mildly, not exactly the most presentable and gregarious of people, the trafficking tradi-tionally fell largely upon the shoulders of the outlaw motorcycle gangs. That changed when the Amezcuas came to town.

"The aggressive and violent nature of Mexican traffickers lit-erally forced the motorcycle groups out of the production business and almost strictly into the mid- to lower-scale distribution," said Kypridakes.

The bikers, for all their bravado and tough-guy image, turned tail and ran when the Mexicans arrived. They continued to work, but only on the fringes and the bottom end of the speed market, serving those markets that weren't profitable enough for the Mexicans to care about.

California is the most populous state in the union, but the Amezcuas were producing more meth than they could sell locally. Suddenly, meth, which had previously been unknown beyond the Pacific Coast, was turning up all over the country, particularly in rural and suburban areas populated predominately or entirely by whites. First it went north to Oregon and Washington, then east. Before 1994 was over, Phoenix had the second-highest rate of meth-related emergency room admissions in the country. San Diego, a California city just across the border from Mexico, remained the leader. The problem was so bad there that, starting in 1994, rehab facilities in San Diego actually started admitting more people for meth than alcohol. And according to the DEA:

> The eastward expansion of the drug took a particular toll on central states such as Arkansas, Illinois, Indiana, Iowa, Kansas, Missouri, and Nebraska. Increased methamphetamine trafficking in these states often in rural areas, is evidenced by a 126 percent increase (1,601 to 3,620) in reported methamphetamine laboratory seizures and an 87 percent increase (10,145 to 18,951) in methamphetamine-related treatment admission. Methamphetamine trafficking has expanded farther east to areas such as southern Michigan, Ohio, and western Pennsylvania.

Later that year, the Clandestine Lab Investigators Association, an organization founded in 1989 by police officers in the western U.S., held their annual conference in Edmonton, Alberta, as meth use had quickly expanded northward to include much of western Canada. Besides the North Americans, officers from England, the Netherlands, Belgium, Poland, Germany, Italy, South Africa, Colombia, Argentina, Thailand and Australia attended—an indication of exactly how widespread meth use had become.

But meth continued to be a phenomenon limited to rural and suburban areas.

"Indianapolis has no meth problem. Six of the nine districts are mostly related to the city of Indianapolis, so that leaves three congressmen out of the nine in Indiana who have a meth problem," said Mark Souder, a Republican member of the House of Representatives from Indiana. "Of those three congressional districts, like mine, the biggest city is Fort Wayne and it has one lab. The rural areas in my district...have a huge meth problem."

"Our methamphetamine started showing up everywhere in the United States," Pennal said. "That's when we realized that we were being used basically as the industrial center. We were basically the Medellín. The way cocaine in Colombia was the Medellín cartel, now we were basically the suppliers for everyone in the United States." He wasn't far off. The DEA's Operation Pipeline in 1993 determined that 92.8 percent of all meth confiscated in the United States could be tracked back to the Golden State.

The meth market was skyrocketing, and the Amezcuas were getting very rich. Contemporary accounts estimated that between 50 and 90 percent of all the meth in the U.S. was manufactured by the cartel. It seemed like nothing could slow them down. But drug trafficking is an unpredictable business. In March 1994, a shipping clerk in Frankfurt faced a dilemma. He had 120 barrel containers in his warehouse destined for Mexico, and the customer wanted them *now*. Everything was going according to plan when the clerk, who asked not be named, received a phone call. It was the airline: bad news. The only flight to Mexico that week was overbooked; his shipment would be bumped. Desperate for an alternative, he found a Lufthansa cargo flight from Switzerland to Mexico that had room to spare. But there was a hitch. The plane was making a stop in Dallas-Fort Worth and his client in Mexico had left express instructions that his cargo was not to be routed through the United States. But, the first rule of shipping is to get it there, and the clerk was pretty sure his client would never know about the detour. He made the call and got the cargo on the plane.

When the cargo landed in Texas, U.S. Customs agents boarded the plane. An officer noticed that the shipping labels had been hastily altered.

"He noticed the company of origin," said Haislip. "You could almost read it through the top cover, but it had been painted over." So he pried off the lid on the first barrel. It didn't surprise the more experienced officers that the powder inside was pure ephedrine. He immediately phoned the DEA, who raced to the scene. The seizure was huge. In total, the Amezcuas lost 3.7 tons of ephedrine or, if it was all used properly, about 41 million hits of meth. At a bargain rate of $10 a dose, that's $410 million. Although ephedrine was legal in the U.S., the shipment wasn't because it wasn't registered with the DEA and the bills of lading had been altered to make it appear as though the barrels contained fertilizer.

"It was a real eye-opener," said Terry Woodworth, who was then the DEA's deputy director of diversion control. "We were, to be candid, not as aware of that situation as we should have been until the Dallas-Fort Worth seizures."

Not only did the authorities make a dent in the amount of ephedrine coming into the U.S. via Mexico, they also found out who it was going to. Of course, the packages didn't give the Amezcuas' names and addresses, but the fact that it was headed for Guadalajara made it pretty clear who would eventually be receiving the powder. Working in conjunction with the Swiss, who actually had no specific laws regarding the import or export of ephedrine but were eager to help stop the production of illegal drugs, the DEA mounted a large-scale international operation. The first targets were the shipping agents. "The brokers didn't really want to deal with us; they didn't want to supply paper; they didn't want to provide information," said Haislip. "But of course we have ways of getting information, and we have ways of getting them to be cooperative."

The investigation revealed that companies in India and the Czech Republic had supplied the Amezcuas with seventy-seven tons of ephedrine, or the equivalent of about 840 million doses of meth—enough to give every man, woman and child in New York City one hundred hits.

Armed with such damning evidence, DEA agents and government officials attended the annual summit held by the International Narcotics Control Board in Vienna and pled their case. After weeks of closed-door negotiations, the Americans managed to hammer out agreements with all of the ephedrine manufacturing countries and many of the authorities who oversaw stopover destinations that serviced Mexico to prevent the sale of ephredrine to the Amezcuas.

It was a severe blow, and not the only one. Haislip's team managed to get a bill passed by Congress in 1996 to force all U.S. ephedrine retailers to register with the DEA, keep products behind the counter and report any suspicious people or transactions. The new law, later known as the Comprehensive Methamphetamine Control Act (MCA), also extended to the transmission of ephedrine and similar chemicals by mail or courier to non-pharmaceutical people.

Earlier, in May 1995, the Internal Revenue Service, acting on information from the DEA, started cracking down on mail-order ephedrine retailers. It was an offensive that took literally millions of pills off the market.

The same year, the DEA seized 33.7 tons of ephedrine and pseudoephedrine they determined were headed for what they called "rogue tablet manufacturers, mail-order distributors and clandestine methamphetamine laboratories."

The repercussions followed quickly. While the average street value of a bottle of one thousand ephedrine pills was generally less than $20 at the end of 1994, it had risen to $385 by the summer of 1995. The price of barrels of ephedrine powder (called "tins" in the industry) started to climb too, but eventually became worthless as word spread in the community that the only people who had them to sell were undercover DEA agents. Purity levels began to fall as well. The average purity level peaked in November 1994 at 74 percent, but fell as low as 40 percent a year later. Perhaps more tellingly, police labs began to find the better part of their confiscated meth was being diluted with methylsulfonylmethane (MSM), a pain reliever that happens to look and taste a lot like meth. Many states, particularly those east of the Mississippi, started recording significant drops in meth-related rehab cases, emergency-room admissions and deaths. Other states reported a slowing of growth in the same statistics for the first time. "We knew that we were having an effect," said Haislip. "We began once again to see that same beautiful fall of the deaths and injuries that tells you you are having success." Investigative newspaper reports from cities that had been overrun by meth, such as Portland, Phoenix, San Diego and Denver, reported significant decreases in petty crimes often associated with meth use such as car theft, forgery, burglary, break and enter, robbery and possession or sale of stolen goods.

According to information the DEA acquired from inform-ants, the Amezcuas held a conference in Tijuana and invited all of their associates to talk about their problems and plan for the future. The police in the Central Valley began to believe they were winning the war in August 1995 when they made a num-ber of busts in which the dealers were selling amphetamines (which can be made without the use of ephedrine) but telling customers it was meth. Clearly, they were desperate.

But that's also about when the DEA's plan hit a snag. Controlling ephedrine wasn't a huge problem. Nobody used ephedrine as a cold remedy. It was a pill used for people desper-ate to lose weight, desperate to drive their tractor-trailer all night or desperate to study enough to be prepared for the exam the next day. Everyone knew it was speed, even before it was transformed into meth. It had a shady reputation and few people were sorry to see it regulated, and those that were often were too scared of being labeled addicts to make much fuss about it. But pseu-doephedrine is another story entirely. Every day, millions of North Americans take pseudoephedrine for their colds and it works, far better than the next-best remedy and with fewer side effects. Although some people are convinced that it's a stimulant and have tried to use it as such, pseudoephedrine by itself actu-ally has little effect on the central nervous system and is generally considered pretty safe to use by the scientific community and public as well. It certainly wasn't ephedrine. Besides, annual legitimate sales of pseudoephedrine tablets figured in the $4-billion range in the U.S. alone. That would be a pretty big slice of pie to wrestle away from the pharmaceutical companies.

And while the MCA covered the sale of powdered pseu-doephedrine, it did nothing to control the sale of pseudoephedrine tablets. This fact was not lost on the meth manufacturers. Soon, sales of cold pills skyrocketed. People, often Mexican nationals, were buying in amounts just small enough to keep the pharmacist from phoning the DEA. They developed a technique called "roller coastering" where individuals who pretended not to know each other arrived at a drugstore at about the same time and all bought the same thing—cold remedies containing pseudoephedrine—then hopped into a van, moved on to another drugstore and repeated the process. At about the same time, legitimate imports of pseudoephedrine tablets to Mexico exploded. While imports had been stable at about thirty tons a year, they suddenly shot up to 224 tons. And that doesn't even account for the millions of tons that Jose Luis Santiago Vasconcelos, Mexico's deputy attorney general for organized crime, admitted were being smuggled to Mexico from other countries, particularly Hong Kong.

While the superlabs were starving for raw materials and meth users were starving for finished product, independent manufacturers began to fill the void. They began to exploit the few advantages they had over the superlabs. In many parts of the U.S. and Canada, there were no Mexicans, let alone those with connections to the Amezcuas or the other cartels—most notably the Tijuana-based Arrellano Felix brothers—that had moved into the business. And, except for parts of California and perhaps Florida, Arizona and Texas, there were very few places in which groups of seemingly non-associated Mexicans could arrive suffering from simultaneous colds without raising suspicion. On the other hand, local people could drive to three or four area drugstores and buy a couple of packages of cold pills from each every few days or so. The men who ran the super labs, always wary of undercover cops, would never buy pills from anyone who wasn't immediately recognized as friends or family, so the people who were buying the pseudoephedrine either had to sell it to the local cook and make their own meth. And, for the first time, they could. Before the middle-Ninetiess, making meth wasn't exactly a closely guarded secret, but it wasn't a widely distributed recipe.

Up until that time, aspiring meth cooks had to learn the trade from experienced chemists or get their hands on one of a few "underground" publications, which were rare. They were distributed only by a few mail-order houses, which were not well known because most other publications refused to carry their ads. But the great democratizing power of the Internet allowed the recipe to be distributed very nearly without limit. Not only were the books more freely available, but people traded information on chat rooms, forums and via e-mail. "In the past, methamphetamine chemists closely guarded their drug recipes," said Donnie R. Marshall, acting chief of the DEA. "But with modern computer technology and the increasing willingness of chemists to share their recipes, this information is now available to anyone with computer access." Suddenly anyone with Internet access, eighty dollars worth of cold pills and household cleaners, a few bottles and hoses and the nerve to risk explosions and chemical burns could go into business making and selling meth.

These new entrepreneurs—though mostly white, blue collar and rural—were no longer being called "redneck labs," but instead became known as "mom 'n' pop labs" or, more frequently, "Beavis and Butt-Head labs," a reference to the two dim-witted cartoon characters who were very popular at the time. It was also an insulting assessment of the dangerously mistake-prone, often less-than-well-educated people who entered the business. "Before you know it, sixty percent of the labs we were dealing with were having fires and explosions," said Pennal. "Because they were learning, and they were making mistakes."

"Well, what happened was that the traditional avenues for meth distribution dried up in a real big hurry," one Missouri-based investigator told me. "So some of the people who wanted, you might say needed, more meth figured out how to make it. We almost forced them to—it was make it yourself or go straight." Police forces that had been seizing one or two labs a year started stumbling upon them in the dozens. Those in California started closing them down in the hundreds. Although the individual labs didn't produce much product, the unprecedented growth in their numbers resulted in an overall growth in meth production and, as more labs started popping up in new places, distribution. According to Marshall, about one-third of the 1600 high school students in Marshalltown, Iowa, had tried meth in 1998.

But the proliferation of labs didn't really make a huge dent in the overall proportion of who was making meth. According to DEA estimates, even at their lowest point, the California super-labs (not all of which were still owned by the Amezcuas as other Mexican-based cartels had established significant operations in the U.S.) were still manufacturing up to 80 percent of all the meth available in the U.S.

The DEA pushed for stricter legislation and what they got what a bizarre compromise. Retail sales of pseudoephedrine would be controlled, except for those tablets that were sold in blister packs—those plastic things where you have to push the pills through foil. The reason behind the decision appeared to be that because it took more time and effort to push pills through blister packs, it was less likely that meth cooks would use them. History, statistics and my own personal observations have proven that this legislation was laughable. At a hearing before the U.S. Senate to determine the best ways to combat meth proliferation, Kypridakes was asked if she had ever run into blister packs at the meth labs she'd visited that had been seized. Her reply was that she had seen "thousands and thousands of the little packages."

The compromise did little to deter the superlabs. The Mexican laborers the cartels employed were more than happy to push pills through foil for barely sustenance wages (it certainly beat picking strawberries) and some enterprising cooks even devised and employed an ingenious purpose-built machine that could be adjusted to different brands. According to a California investigator I spoke with, "they had two settings, Sudafed and Contac-C." That thousandth of a millimeter of aluminum did precious little to stop the people determined to make meth. At jumping off points on the Mexican side of the U.S. border, there are fields full of thousands of piled-up boxes that had once contained cold pills.

And the cartels began to get smarter about skirting the controls on pseudoephedrine powder, avoiding suppliers who had spoken with the DEA and finding new ones. Haislip and his crew kept chasing them, but the cartels always seemed to find someone new would will sell them powder. They would also form shell companies in various countries, acquiring the chemical legally and then smuggling it into California. And simple bribery and other means of coercion helped open up supply lines from legitimate retailers, particularly in East Los Angeles and Oakland.

Meth not only changed the United States and Canada, but Mexico as well. Although it's probably best known for the millions of monarch butterflies which migrate there every year, the cool, humid winds that blow across the plateaus in the southern state of Michoacan have long made it famous as the best farmland in the country. Traditionally, farmers have grown some of the world's best watermelons, papayas, tomatoes and especially mangoes. More recently, however, Michoacan has become better known for its marijuana. Treasured by aficionados, weed from Michoacan is prized for its strength and is said to be freer of contaminants than most. Other enterprising Michoacanos have repurposed many of the higher, more secluded fields for the cultivation of highly lucrative opium poppies.

Perhaps it was their long and successful experience as drug suppliers that gave them a reputation as experts among their fellow Mexicans, but Michoacan, especially the small city of Apatzignan, traditionally supplied most of the cooks employed by the superlabs. "Oh yeah, whenever we arrest a guy and we suspect he's a cook, we ask him if he's from Apatzignan," one California drug officer told me. "It seems like they all are." It's not a coincidence. "It's like they have some kind of mini-academy down there in Apatzignan where they train people to cook and send them to California," said Mike Huerta, a Phoenix-based DEA agent. It's a widely held opinion, although nobody has ever found Meth Cook U.

But if you go to Apatzignan, you can see the effects of its playing host to the school. Like most southern Mexican towns, it radiates from the old town and the streets are lined with shops—often nothing more than a blanket covered in pro-duce—crowds of young men talking and joking with one another and equally large groups of young women with baby strollers. But what separates Apatzignan from its neighbors is that every bit of paved road is occupied by a big-buck German sedan, American SUV or, the most desired of all, a customized Chevy, Ford or Dodge pickup. The more chrome, the better. All of these vehicles are piloted by young men splashed with jewelry and painted with tattoos. And while American hip-hop rumbles out of some, most blast a constant soundtrack of narcocorridos.

Played with guitars and accordions and set to a polka-like beat, corridos are part of the Mexican folk music tradition. Their lyrics often tell of real events in a romantic fashion and many have been written and sung about folk heroes like Pancho Villa and his exploits. Narcocorridos, as the name suggests, typically tell stories of drug smugglers, cooks and dealers crossing the border into the United States, striking it rich and returning home as heroes or dying in the attempt. The similarity to "old-skool" gangsta rap is not coincidental. Not surprisingly, government, advocacy groups and media organizations have tried (largely in vain) to ban narcocorridos from radio and television. But it wouldn't make much of a difference if what fans of the music tell me is true. The music has become a weird soundtrack for a new kind of cult hro: Robin Hood meets Tupak. Certain words and phrases are banned, so the artists simply substitute slang terms their audiences know, but the feds don't.

It's all a pretty strong advertisement for the business. As Apatzignan police officer Ramon Lopez-Valencia told an American reporter: "It's true—all the young people want to be crystal dealers."

But for all its wealth, Apatzignan has acquired a new problem—locals are now beginning to use meth. And there have been obvious escalations in the problems associated with it, like health problems and crime. "Crystal is a gigantic problem here," said the town's police chief, Fernando Fernandez-Castaneda. "We used to take it all out of the country, but now the locals are consuming it and it's very worrisome." While it may be tempting for a cook to sample his wares, it's not that common. Aspiring cooks are repeatedly informed that no addict has a chance at a job in an American superlab, and that's what they're there for. Instead, it's the mules who smuggle the drugs or simply rank-and-file Mexicans who begin to use. "I think there's so much available, so cheaply, that that's how poor people in Mexico are able to obtain it," said Suo. "In many cases, the cartels will pay mules in drugs, as opposed to in cash. So that's why some experts think that meth has become particularly a problem in border towns like Tijuana."

The Mexicans, pressured by the DEA, made significant progress in tracking the cartels and in the early morning hours of June 1, 1998, heavily armed officers from their anti-drug agency, Fiscalia Especial Para Atencion a los Delitos Contra la Salud (FEADS), descended upon the home of Luis Ignacio Amezcua-Contreras' girlfriend and arrested him inside. On the following day, Jose de Jesus Amezcua-Contreras was arrested on the road heading out of Guadalajara. (He was discovered hiding in the trunk of a car being driven in the direction of Colima, their hometown.) The brothers were sent to the same federal maximum-security prison in Mexico City that held their younger brother Adan and their brother-in-law Jaime Ladino. Both of them had been arrested in the previous year in Colima; Adan on weapons charges and Ladino for drug trafficking.

At the time, the DEA was ecstatic. "The Amezcua brothers run the largest methamphetamine and chemical trafficking organization identified by U.S. law enforcement, and the arrest and removal of these two key leaders should significantly disrupt the established methamphetamine trade which is carried out by organized crime leaders in Mexico," said DEA Administrator Thomas A. Constantine. "DEA shares with the Government of Mexico the goal of completely destroying this organization and any others like it."

Although it was estimated at the time that the Amezcuas controlled up to three-quarters of the meth business in the U.S., Constantine's optimism was short-lived. Within weeks, Luis and Jesus were released due to (as is commonplace when rich and powerful people are indicted in Mexico) "lack of evidence." They were, however, picked up again days later after the U.S. State Department pointed out that there were outstanding warrants for their arrest by American authorities. In January, a court ruled that the brothers were extraditable, but they remained in prison while the two countries haggled over what was to be done with them. Adan, however, walked when a judge ruled that there was a "lack of evidence" to convict him.

There's a difference of opinion as to who runs the Amezcua cartel now. Some say it's Luis and Jesus' sisters and others have told me that it's this or that brother-in-law. But none deny that it's still alive and thriving. Still, news of the brothers' arrests sent a shockwave of opportunity through Mexico. Many believed that the Amezcuas were finished, so still other cartels moved in and set up new, or strengthened existing, operations. Meth production, purity and indications of use actually grew after the brothers were arrested.

As the number of meth users and meth-related crimes began to rise again, authorities in the U.S. began to look for other answers. Pfizer, the largest pharmaceutical firm in the world and the makers of Sudafed, began to work on chemical strains of pseudoephedrine that could not be made into meth. After spending about $25 million and years of research to develop such a product, the company gave up. "The tough lesson that we learned is, as fast as we could do things, following all of the rules—the FDA guidelines and things that make drugs appropriately safe—well, the meth cooks could move a lot more quickly," said Steve Robins, group marketing director for Pfizer. "So every time we would try to create an enhancement that would block them, they changed their process so they could extract it."

In 2000, the DEA cracked down on black market pseudoephedrine sales and arrested a number of pharmacists, assistants, warehouse employees and other people with access to the pills. But, to their surprise, the purity of street-level meth continued to rise, as did the key indicators of meth use like emergency room visits, rehab admissions and petty crimes. That's when it became apparent that the superlabs were getting their raw materials from another direction—this time from the north. In 2000 and 2001, officers seizing meth labs began to notice that many of the cold pill boxes they found on scene had French on their labels. Before long, tons of pseudoephedrine pills started being confiscated at border crossings into the U.S. from Canada. With no meaningful regulations in place governing the sale of pseudoephedrine, Canadian pharmacies experienced a boom in sales, as imports of the drug jumped from about thirty-seven tons in 2000 to just over 154 tons in 2001. "It was clear that a significant portion of the methamphetamine traffickers and manufacturers had turned to that source of supply," said Haislip. "Canada was a weak link. Canada had a weak law. Canada really wasn't giving attention to this, and it was well-known." Ironically, both American and Canadian authorities linked the purchase and transportation of pseudoephedrine from Canada to the Hells Angels and other outlaw motorcycle gangs. While some of their business was with the small labs, the bulk of it was believed to be with the Mexican superlabs. In just a few short years, the bikers went from dominating the meth market to being supplanted by the Mexicans to serving as their vassals.

Adan Amezcua-Contreras was arrested on money-laundering charges in May 2001 and thrown into the same prison that held Luis and Jesus. About a year later, a Mexican judge ruled against the extradition of the Amezcuas because the U.S. could not guarantee that they would not face life imprisonment. Mexican law quite clearly states that the country will not extradite any suspect who is likely to receive a life sentence or the death penalty. Although they remain in prison, the cartel is believed to be operating well without them and there are some people who maintain that they still have at least some say in the organization's day-to-day operations.

In 2003, the Canadian government passed the Control of Precursor and Other Substances Frequently Used in the Clandestine Production of Controlled Substances Act, which established regulations regarding pseudoephedrine that were similar to those in place in the U.S.

Perhaps more important, the Royal Canadian Mounted Police (RCMP) began to monitor suspected pseudoephedrine smugglers and work in conjunction with the DEA to arrest them on both sides of the border. Later that year, law enforcement from both countries launched Operation North Star, an attempt to target and bring down Canada's illegal pseudoephedrine imports. Large-scale arrests were made in ten Canadian cities and major charges were laid against three pharmaceutical companies. One of the most important ones occurred on April 8, 2003, when the RCMP and the Integrated National Security Enforcement Team—a group made up of officers from other federal, provincial and local agencies—raided a warehouse in Richmond, a suburb of Vancouver. Not only did they find ten million pseudoephedrine tablets mislabeled and headed for the U.S., they also found enough evidence to indict six executives from three legitimate Quebec-based pharmaceutical companies for knowingly supplying clandestine labs with the raw materials necessary for the manufacture of illegal drugs. More Canadians on the scene were arrested on warrants from U.S. authorities and the RCMP also confiscated $1.6 million in U.S. currency and a top-of-the-line SUV. "We believe that Operation Northern Star has disrupted a major pseudoephedrine pipeline from Canada and sent a clear message to pharmaceutical companies there and elsewhere that they will be held criminally responsible for dispensing their products in the United States for illegal use," said then-U.S. Assistant Attorney General Michael Chertoff.

But as the RCMP was cracking down on exports of pseudoephedrine, Canadian use of meth skyrocketed. While the feds seized just two labs in Canada in 1998, that number rose to thirty-seven in 2003. Over the same time period, the number of meth-related deaths in the Western province of British Columbia climbed from three to thirty-three. As in the U.S., Canadian officials began to see significant spikes in the types of crimes associated with meth (especially car thefts) when the drug became established in their communities. According both to officers and dealers I have spoken with, many Canadians in the pseudoephedrine export business were actually paid in meth. It was an astute plan and one taken right out of the Amezcuas' play-book. The key to successful retailing is repeat business and who comes back more faithfully than an addict? Getting people hooked on meth guaranteed the existence of a domestic market. And, as had happened in the U.S. earlier, meth spread through-out the country as outlaw motorcycle gangs (which are still firmly at the top of the organized crime food chain in Canada), Asian crime rings and other groups introduced the low-cost, high profit stimulant to their traditional menu of marijuana, hashish, cocaine and prostitution. "It's right across the country now," Scott Rintoul, the RCMP's drug awareness coordinator in Vancouver, said of meth. "In Toronto and Montreal and the east coast, it's there now—it may not be at the same level as here, but it's definitely moving from west to east."

The restrictions may have had a profound effect on the amount of pseudoephedrine available in the United States from Canada, but did little to reduce the amount of meth on the streets. The World Health Organization even issued a press release stating that meth had become "the most widely used illicit drug after marijuana." Ever adaptable, the Mexican cartels gradually moved their production from the Central Valley in California to the Guadalajara area of western Mexico. Instead of smuggling pseudoephedrine over the Rio Grande, they started carrying meth. Sure the penalties were higher, but it was only the mules who were taking the risk.

The result was that meth use grew. In 2003, a survey of state and local law enforcement departments revealed that 91 percent of those in the Pacific region identified meth as their primary drug problem. So the feds came up with a plan. On October 25, 2004, John Walters (officially the director of National Drug Control Policy for the President's Office of National Drug Control Policy, but better known as the nation's "Drug Czar") and DEA administrator Karen Tandy announced the National

Synthetic Drugs Action Plan, an outline of how the federal government planned to combat meth (along with other purpose-made drugs like ecstasy) and help out the people and places it had affected. Although it's a long and complicated document, the key elements to keep in mind was that it meant more money for enforcement and stiffer sentences for those convicted of related offenses.

But the feds were only doing what the states had already started. Six months earlier, Oklahoma passed a law that limited the amount of pseudoephedrine pharmacies could buy, forced them to keep the tablets (foil pack or not) behind the counter and to require buyers to show identification and sign a register. A similar law had been defeated in Oregon some years earlier, but by the time the National Synthetic Drugs Action Plan was announced, twenty-three states had some law on the books that in some way limited or restricted the retail sale of pseudoephedrine.

That total grew to thirty-five by the time 2005 arrived. After hearing arguments from politicians from the districts and states worst affected by meth and also from the lobbyists employed by the pharmaceutical industry, Congress passed the Combat Methamphetamine Epidemic Act of 2005 as part of a far-reaching set of laws called the Patriot Act. It stipulates, among other things, that retailers must keep pseudoephedrine behind locked doors and that the registers buyers sign be made available to the federal government. It also earmarked more money and manpower to help meth and precursor drug investigations in Mexico, Canada and, to a lesser extent, other countries. Walters' replacement as Drug Czar, Scott M. Burns, testified:

> In sixteen years as a prosecutor in a rural [Utah] county,
> I learned about the destructive nature of methamphetamine first-hand by working frequently with police

officers who were put at risk by having to respond to, enter and 'sit on' methamphetamine labs; by meeting with innocent neighbors who lived near houses turned into methamphetamine labs; and by discovering children whose parents were found to be under the influence of methamphetamine, and suffered neglect as a result. Methamphetamine is undeniably a uniquely destructive drug.

After its lack of success trying to alter pseudoephedrine so that it could not be used as a meth precursor, Pfizer simply switched chemicals. In January 2005 it introduced Sudafed PE to the U.S. and Canadian markets after it had been on sale for a little more than a year in Europe. Instead of pseudoephedrine, the new drug's active ingredient was phenylephrine, which can't be made into meth by any technique. Actually, phenylephrine had been on the market for years, usually taken in the form of a lemon-flavored hot drink (known as Neo-Citran in Canada and LemSip in the U.K.) or a nasal spray, often called Neosynephrine. And, as more than four thousand products containing pseudoephedrine were on the U.S. market, big pharmaceutical firms offered remedies with phenylephrine like Bayer's Alka-Seltzer Cold Effervescent Formula and Vicks' DayQuil capsules as an alternative.

Phenylephrine is generally considered less effective than pseudoephedrine and there's actually some debate whether it even works at all. It has a problem with first-pass metabolism (meaning that the body often digests the drug, preventing it from entering the bloodstream and having any medicinal effect) and according to a study authored by Dr. Leslie Hendeles, professor of pharmacy and pediatrics at the University of Florida's Colleges of Pharmacy and Medicine, "phenylpropanolamine and pseudoephedrine, but not phenylephrine, are effective decongestants." If you're wondering why Pfizer didn't choose phenylpropanolamine instead, it's because it was removed from the market in 2001 after it was positively linked to hemorrhagic stroke. While people can argue over which drug is more efficient or easier to take than the others, traditionally phenylephrine ran a distant third in sales behind pseudoephedrine and oxymetazoline, the active ingredient in Vicks' Sinex products and a chemical that has a distinct history of becoming habit-forming. Part of the public's reluctance to switch to phenylephrine may also have been its side effects, which can include nausea, hallucinations and an irregular heartbeat. A significant number of people can experience allergic reactions to the drug and it is not recommended for anyone who could have hypertension or diabetes.

Pfizer didn't replace Sudafed with Sudafed PE; it just offered the new remedy as an alternative. "Original Sudafed will still be available, but where sales of pseudoephedrine are restricted or placed 'behind the counter,' Sudafed PE will provide consumers with a convenient 'on-the-shelf' decongestant," Jay Kominsky, Pfizer's vice chairman, said.

Suddenly, politicians and advocates piled on. Since phenylephrine had been around for decades, many wondered aloud why Pfizer simply hadn't replaced pseudoephedrine with it and done so earlier.

"It seems fairly clear that Sudafed as a brand is a cash cow for Pfizer," said Paul Laymon, assistant U.S. attorney for Chattanooga, Tenn., and an expert at prosecuting meth cases. "I could understand why they would want to protect their flagship brand. Are their decisions motivated by profit? It would seem pretty obvious that it is."

Pfizer's official response was that they didn't discontinue their pseudoephedrine products because people knew and trusted them and that government limitations were designed to keep it out of the hands of those who would abuse it. The timing, they said, was designed to coincide with the successful conclusion of their efforts to ensure that the pseudoephedrine in their products could not be repurposed for the meth industry.

"It is a long and painstakingly difficult process, the reformulation," said Elizabeth Assey, a spokeswoman for Consumer Healthcare Products Association, a Washington-based trade association made up of suppliers of over-the-counter medicines. "We believe our member companies have worked in earnest at ways to provide alternatives. Our members don't want to see their products ending up in the meth labs."

Interestingly, Schering-Plough, which makes Claritin-D and is Pfizer's biggest rival in the cold remedy business, and McNeil Consumer and Specialty Pharmaceuticals, which makes Tylenol and Motrin products, announced no plans for pseudoephedrine alternatives and also continued to fight against forcing their products behind the counter.

A few months later, in November, the Mexican government announced that it would play ball. Almost immediately after the U.S. House of Representatives voted 432-2 for a bill that contained a certification clause that would slash American aid to any country that imported too much of the precursor chemicals for methamphetamine, the Mexican government announced a sweeping plan to reduce pseudoephedrine imports and their illegal use. It was an interesting piece of legislation, actually. The U.S. government would examine official pseudoephedrine imports and exports from the countries in question and compare them to a battery of statistics including population, climate, medical facilities and how much of the chemical they handled before the meth epidemic. Part of the evidence presented included the fact that Canada, which does not manufacture pseudoephedrine, sent twelve tons of the chemical to Panama in 2004, a country where few colds are suffered but happens to be on the Colombia-to-Mexico drug pipeline. Perhaps tellingly, Panama had received just 1.7 tons from all sources the year before. Also cited was the fact that Montserrat, a tiny hurricane- and volcano-ravaged island in the Caribbean, received 2.2 tons of pseudoephedrine in 2004, apparently to counter the sniffles of its 4488 people. For a sun-drenched nation with no actual factories or pharmacies, legally importing a shade more than two pounds of cold medicine for every person on the island raises a few suspicions.

In what was officially a change of heart and a desire to curb the meth menace, Mexican ambassador to the U.S. Carlos de Icaza told Congress that Mexico would slash its pseudoephedrine imports to 1999 levels—about fifty-one tons or less than a quarter of their 2004 imports. He also announced that only licensed drug stores with a full-time pharmacist would be allowed to sell pseudoephedrine, reducing the number of retail outlets from 51,000 to 17,000. This was a big turnaround from the days (literally days) earlier when Vasconcelos, basically the top drug enforcement agent in Mexico, denied in an interview with an American newspaper that Mexican pseudoephedrine was a significant part of what he called "America's meth problem."

The reaction north of the Rio Grande was predictable.

"This is an important step forward, which I hope will signal a new cooperation on fighting the meth epidemic," said Feinstein. Others were less political and more direct.

"It would be wrong and presumptuous of us to assume that the only reason they would do this is that we have a certification provision in the bill," said Brian Baird, a Democratic congressman from Washington and one of the founders of the "Meth Caucus," a group of politicians from the methamphetamine-affected areas of the country. "By the same token, I think putting that in the bill sends a pretty strong message. And frankly, if they're doing these kinds of things, I don't think they should have a great fear about certification." Although he has a point, it still seems like a pretty chilling thing for a politician to say. While it may seem conveniently ironic to some who like that sort of thing, the U.S. itself has no official quotas on the amount of pseudoephedrine that it may import, other controls have brought per-capita imports in line with other large Western economies.

In the summer of 2006, the World Health Organization determined that meth was the most widely used "hard drug" in the world with 26 million users, including 1.4 million in the U.S. but with the majority of the remainder in Southeast Asia. If you believe the WHO's numbers, there are more meth users on our planet than cocaine and heroin users put together. In their official 2004 report on the management of substance abuse, the WHO had very little good news regarding speed, which they refer to as "ATS," which stands for "amphetamine-type stimulants:"

> For many countries, the problem of ATS is relatively new, growing quickly and unlikely to go away. The geographical spread is widening, but awareness of it is limited and responses are neither integrated nor consistent.... There are about twenty countries in which the abuse of ATS is more widespread than that of heroin and cocaine combined. Japan, Korea and the Philippines all register five to seven times the rate of ATS use compared with heroin and cocaine use.... The present situation warrants immediate attention, with a major epidemic of methamphetamine use in Thailand that appears to be spreading across the entire Asia-Pacific region.

In spite of the national and international controls of precursor chemicals and the increased pressure on cooks, distributors and users by law enforcement, most places and the world in general are seeing an increase, sometimes meteoric, in the signs of meth use.

Maybe Gene Haislip, the DEA cop who successfully battled the American Quaalude market, was right. Maybe if the DEA had managed to control pseudoephedrine in the same way it had methaqualone, phenyl-2-propanone and ephedrine, then meth would have been snuffed out before it became a large-scale epidemic. Maybe, but it's probably too late.

BEATING THE TEST

TestClear is an Oklahoma City-based company that specializes in helping people pass drug tests (although they also sell hangover pills and semen-detecting "infidelity tests"). With the stated purpose "to help individuals and their families achieve a better standard of living based on their knowledge, skills, abilities, and not on their lifestyle," TestClear offers a number of different products to help the meth user test negative. Here's a representative sample with TestClear's sales pitch (prices are in U.S. dollars and were accurate for July 2006):

Powdered Urine Kit: The powdered urine kit is the only proven solution recommend for a job or insurance situation because it has never failed and you don't have to quit to pass the test. $43.95

Klear Urine Additive: Klear is an additive that is not recommended for use in the United States. We have heard of good success stories in Europe and Canada. $30.00

Mega Clean Cleansing Drink: When your situation is critical and you can't afford not to be clean Mega Clean is the product for you. Mega Clean is the Cadillac of drink products with free PreCleanse Pills and double money back guarantee. $75.95

SpitNKleen Mouthwash: For a Saliva Test is the most effective product that we have found. If you are faced with a swab or saliva test this is the product for you. Guaranteed to work or your money back. $47.95

Saliva Drug Testing Kit: Know before you go! Tests for amphetamine, methampetamine, marijuana, PCP, cocaine, and opiates in the saliva. Uses the same cutoff as recommended by the federal government. $29.95

Source: TestClear.com

MR. SCIENCE:
THIS IS YOUR BRAIN
ON METH

Brain CHEMISTRY IS hard to understand. But to put it into an easy-to-understand perspective, take a look at a more simplified version of an adult—a baby (if you don't have a baby, an even simpler version, a dog, will also work). Spending some time with either, you'll notice that there are two ways to make them happy. The first is stimulation, or becoming excited. Play peek-a-boo with the baby (or fetch with the dog) and you'll see unfettered delight. The baby will smile, squeal and give every possible indication of enjoyment. Unless, that it is, you keep it up for too long. There's only so much stimulus a brain can take. Go too far in your game of peek-a-boo (you'll find the dog harder to overstimulate) and you'll see indications of anxiety, fear and even anger from the baby. An overstimulated baby quickly becomes a crying, yowling mess.

But there is a cure for overstimulation and it's also the other way to make a brain happy. By removing the stimulus and replacing it with comfort, the crying will stop. Pick the baby up, hug it, cuddle it, keep it warm and take it away from light and noise and it will become happy again. Don't be surprised if it falls asleep. Ironically, the other way to get happy, what we might call relaxing, is the exact opposite of excitement.

WHEN WE HAD health class in high school, they'd take out the girls and combine two boys' classes. I think the official reasoning was that it allowed students of both sexes to discuss personal health-related issues with less anxiety, but I'm pretty sure it was because the teachers felt more comfortable dealing with same-sex classes. During a segment on the dangers of drug abuse, one of our teachers was giving a lecture on alcohol. I was daydreaming when something Mr. Muirhead said woke me up. He was explaining the effects of alcohol and told the collection of bored teenagers that alcohol was a depressant. Without thinking, I shouted out "no it isn't!"

Although I got the laugh, I also got a tennis ball in the back of the head from Mr. Brown, who was patrolling the back of the class, ever vigilant, looking for troublemakers such as me so he could whip his tennis ball of discipline at the offender. It's just the way things happened back in the 1980s. A friend of mine got the same treatment when he commented on the "skankiness" of an actress in a film we were shown about sexually transmitted diseases, only he actually got knocked out of his chair.

The guys in class either knew or pretended to know what I was talking about. A depressant? He must be nuts or, as we all expected, a liar. Most of us guys were already at least social drinkers and we knew from experience that it didn't make us depressed at all. In fact, it had the opposite effect, it made most of us happier than we had ever been before. Our shared moment of insurrection came from the fact that we considered alcohol anything but depressing. But while Mr. Muirhead wasn't actually lying, he was being a little misleading.

Alcohol is one of a family of drugs called depressants, like barbiturates and narcotics, but they don't depress us in that they make us feel bad (at least not at first). The name is derived from the fact that they depress or, if you prefer, suppress some of our brain activity. Taking a depressant triggers many of the same reactions as relaxing. Just as the baby cradled in your arm or the dog curled up at your feet feel good, taking a depressant can put you in a mood very much like that glorious state of well-being you generally only experience just as you are drifting off to sleep. But while we are enjoying that blissful feeling, we also suffer some other somnambulant symptoms like slurred speech, a lack of coordination, blurred or double vision and dizziness.

The process is fairly simple. Brain activity generally happens when messages travel across any of the 100 trillion to 1 quadrillion synapses—tiny gaps between brain cells—in our heads. The spaces between the cells are too wide for electrical impulses to jump, so they must be carried by a chemical—usually a hormone. These synapses are firing all the time with various impulses and must be suppressed occasionally, not just to allow us to rest and sleep, but to prevent hallucinations and psychosis.

The hormone that calms us down, lets us relax, puts us to sleep and keeps us sane is gamma-aminobutyric acid (better known as GABA). There's a long and complicated explanation as to how it works, but the upshot is that GABA is the hormone that makes us feel good by slowing everything down and putting a stop to all the hormones that make us feel bad.

Alcohol, like other depressants, binds to the GABA receptors in synapses, allowing GABA to flow more efficiently and with greater amounts in many different parts of the brain. That's why alcohol affects so many parts of the body, from the wobbly legs to the blurred vision to the tongue that sometimes feels too big for your mouth. Among the impulses GABA, and alcohol, suppress are our inhibitions, the self-limiters that prevent us, when sober, from doing what we happily do when we're drunk. "GABA is an inhibitory neurotransmitter," said Kim Fromme, professor of psychology at the University of Texas in Austin. "When activated by alcohol, GABA is thought to contribute to the anxiety reduction and relaxation many people experience from alcohol."

As great as that sounds, there are drawbacks, and they are more severe than hangovers. Unfortunately, human brains are a bit lazy. When someone is doing their job for them, they sort of forget how to do it themselves. Prolonged and heavy usage of alcohol inhibits the brain's ability to bind GABA, which deprives the brain of the precious hormone. The result is that when the brain is deprived of alcohol, the addict (which we normally call an alcoholic) experiences insomnia, jitteriness, anxiety, anger, real depression and tremors. If the addiction is bad enough, you can add convulsions and even death to the list.

STIMULANTS, LIKE METH, work in something of a different way, and with the opposite effect. Instead of GABA, stimulants increase the flow of different transmitting neurohormones—primarily dopamine, norepinephrine, and serotonin—to the synapses.

Dopamine is primarily associated with pleasure—although some scientists differ, saying that it is more involved with desire, the precursor of pleasure—and can be triggered normally by things like food, sex or companionship. But it also has other duties, including giving the body the ability to make smooth coordinated movements. A lack of dopamine has been associated with Parkinson's disease, in which the affected person loses the ability to make smooth movements or stop trembling. Dopamine also allows for clear thought, and the lack of it is thought to contribute to attention deficit disorder and schizophrenia.

Similarly, norepinephrine regulates blood pressure, heart rate and the sugar level in the blood in order to sharpen focus, quicken reactions and increase the confidence in one's own opinions and decisions. Also known as the fight-or-flight response, norepinephrine reactions also increase muscle readiness and can actually convert fat into energy. When released in large amounts, norepinephrine not only makes us more capable in emergency situations, it makes everything an emergency. One byproduct of that effect is that it removes much of the brain's decision-making process away from the conscious mind and gives it over to the more instinctual parts.

The third neurohormone, serotonin, plays a huge part in the regulation of mood, sexuality, hunger and sleep. Too much serotonin dials up the mood and the sex drive and pushes back appetite and the need for sleep. It's also a powerful vasoconstrictor, meaning that it squeezes the blood vessels, increasing blood pressure, internal temperature and loosening the nasal passages.

All of these neurotransmitters and GABA occur naturally in the brain and generally maintain some kind of equilibrium, which determines much of the brain owner's personality. Of course, different sets of stimuli (what we might call situations) evoke the production of different neurotransmitters. If a train is speeding at you, your brain will pump out what it feels is enough norepinephrine to get you out of the way in time. If you're in bed after a satisfying day of work, a good meal and a long bath, your GABA is going to be flowing freely.

After the stimulus is removed, the neurotransmitters aren't very useful—once you've gotten out of the way of the speeding train, there's very little need for norepinephrine—and are removed in a process called reuptake. In reuptake, excess hormones are absorbed back into the brain. Although that's the natural way the brain works, sometimes doctors try to improve the process. When some people need more serotonin because they are depressed, they may be prescribed selective serotonin reuptake inhibitors (SSRIS). These drugs—like Prozac and Xanax—slow down serotonin reuptake when appropriate, leaving more serotonin in the brain and giving some very effective relief from depression.

Cocaine and other stimulants work in much the same way, but in a much larger magnitude. There's no selectiveness and it's not just serotonin. Until the cocaine is totally metabolized by the body, reuptake is turned off for dopamine, norepinephrine and serotonin. Pools of the hormones build up and take effect on the brain. With all of those chemicals raging, the coke users feel strong, confident, bold and sexy. They don't feel a need to eat or sleep. It's a great feeling, as long as it lasts.

As effective as cocaine is, methamphetamine has a couple of advantages over it, even when compared to crack. The first is that it takes much longer to metabolize, staying in the body for twelve to fifteen hours, as opposed to thirty to 120 minutes for the same amount of cocaine. The other is that methamphetamine doesn't just prevent the reuptake of neurotransmitters, but also stimulates the production of dopamine. While cocaine leaves the brain wading in pools of hormones, meth sends it surfing on waves of them. "Synaptic levels of dopamine increase by seven-hundred to twelve-hundred percent after an intoxicating dose of ice," said Dr. Mary Holley, founder of Mothers Against Meth. "It's like you took the lid off a fire hydrant and all the water came rushing out." Those levels of dopamine (not to mention the other hormones involved) could never be achieved without drugs, which is why meth users are almost always at a loss to describe the high. There's simply no frame of reference for people who haven't tried it.

There are problems with it, though. All that dopamine can result in the creation of a few unwanted elements. "The increased presence of dopamine in the extravesicular area of the terminal results in the formation of free radicals," said UCLA'S

Rawson. "It is believed that these free radicals are one of the primary causes of the destruction of the presynaptic dopamine terminals." Free radicals are molecules that emerge because of rapid-fire and uncontrolled reactions with oxygen in the body. They end up with an odd number of electrons which makes them prone to quick bonding. When they bond with other cells, they can damage or even destroy them and, once bonding has begun, can create a domino effect in which whole areas of the brain are affected. The brain has a natural defense for free radicals called antioxidants, which are designed to bond with the free radicals before they can damage cells. But if there are more free radicals than antioxidants, they bond with and hurt or kill the hormone receptors connected to the synapses. As synaptic receptors become damaged or destroyed, the user loses brain power. This phenomenon contributes to the concept of the "burnt out" drug user who has a hard time putting together complex thoughts or accessing even the most ingrained memories.

But far more hurtful than the free radicals are the high levels of dopamine. Under normal circumstances, when dopamine is released and then reabsorbed, there is a period during which the brain has to go without the hormone while it makes more. Ordinarily, this dopamine "fast" isn't noticeable because other hormones take over and establish a different kind of equilibrium. For example, after a stressful but enjoyable experience—like a tennis game—when dopamine is flowing, there's a lack of it afterward. But you don't feel bad because the GABA and other hormones take over, perhaps egged on by a couple of post-match beers, and you experience relaxation.

It doesn't work that way with meth. Neurons aren't like voluntary muscle cells; exercise doesn't make them stronger. The cells that produce and transmit dopamine quickly become overwhelmed by the unnaturally huge amounts they have to deal with. And they lose the ability to make or handle the hormone and die in great numbers. And the receptors suffer, too. Built to receive small to moderate amounts of dopamine, receptors can easily be damaged or destroyed by the excessive amounts triggered by meth. The simile I've heard most often likens the receptor to a human ear—normal dopamine reception is like listening to music, sometimes too soft, occasionally a bit loud, while the same process on meth is like having your ear pressed up against a jet engine. Although the cells are designed to handle dopamine—as ears comprehend sound—they can be overwhelmed and die in large numbers when exposed to excessive amounts. "Methamphetamine has been shown to be neurotoxic to dopamine terminals when administered to laboratory animals, including monkeys," said Rawson.

After even just a few doses, meth users can damage or destroy a number of their dopamine makers, transmitters and receivers.

"Chronic methamphetamine users have a significant loss of dopamine transporters (used as markers of the dopamine terminal) that are associated with slower motor function and decreased memory," said Rawson. "Studies using positron emission tomography have found that methamphetamine-dependent users demonstrate a significantly lower level of dopamine receptors compared to non-drug abusing controls."

Although scientists anticipated the fact that meth would have a significant effect on brain tissue, few were prepared for what they saw the first time a user's brain was image-mapped. "We expected some brain changes but didn't expect so much tissue to be destroyed," said Paul Thompson, associate professor at UCLA's Lab of Neuro Imaging and the first person to gauge the loss of brain power in meth users. "It was shocking, it was like a forest fire of brain damage."

Most affected among meth users tested was the limbic region, a portion of the deepest center of the brain, which controls mood, reward and emotion. According to Thompson, those "cells are dead and gone." That explains why frequent users are depressed and unmoved by the things that normally make us happy.

"Oh sure, I know what they're talking about," said Julie, a long-time meth user with whom I discussed the doctors' opinions. "Before the meth, I cared about everything; afterwards I didn't even care about my own kids."

Almost as affected as the limbic region are the hippocampi, the parts of the brain that control general memory, spatial memory and the ability to navigate. Studies by the researchers at UCLA showed that people who have used meth long enough show many of the same symptoms as people with Alzheimer's disease. According to Thompson, long-term meth users scored much lower on memory tests than healthy people with the same attributes. "One thing the drug users reported was loss of memory," he said. "They have poorer memory than people of the same age and the loss of tissue in the memory areas of the brain is linked to this functional decline. So, people who lost most tissue in the memory areas actually had worse performance on tasks that involved memory."

At first, this phenomenon expresses itself as longer and harsher hangovers. But then it gets more depressing. The remaining dopamine-related cells become weak and dependent on the drug.

As meth use continues, not only does the ability to produce dopamine decrease, but so does the ability to appreciate it. Before long, things that had been previously satisfying—dinner, a movie, sex or taking care of your child—become insufficient. The amount of dopamine produced by activities not related to meth no longer registers in the ailing brain, your steak begins to taste like cardboard and sex might as well be doing push-ups. Meth becomes addictive not just for the normal, chemical reasons, but because there is simply no happiness without it. It's impossible for a non-addict to truly comprehend it, but if you take enough meth, nothing else ever feels good. "You get to the point where it's like if it doesn't taste good or feel good, why bother?' said Justin, a long-time meth user from rural southern Ontario. "Instead of eating or doing whatever, you just think about your next taste and how you're going to get it." And sadly, as it destroys more and more of the brain that handles good feelings, even meth itself gets less potent. So, in order to counter the creeping feeling of depression and nothingness, users find themselves taking bigger doses of methamphetamine more often.

Of course, what meth does for dopamine, it also does for other neurotransmitters, especially serotonin. One of the primary duties of serotonin is to regulate when we sleep. Without sufficient amounts of it, meth addicts never really grow tired until the drug wears off. Binge users may go without sleep for three or four days. Staying up that long usually results in irritability, blurred vision, slurred speech, memory lapses, nausea, confusion, hallucinations and psychosis.

"When people take crystal meth and become dependent on the drug, there is a real change in how the brain works," said Edythe London, a neuroscientist from UCLA. "Very specifically, those circuits in the brain that are primarily in the pre-frontal cortex are down-regulated." The pre-frontal cortex is the part of the brain that controls what's called executive function, which gives us (among other things) the ability to predict outcomes and make appropriate decisions based on them. Without a properly functioning pre-frontal cortex, long-term meth users no longer have the ability to match cause with probable effect. With this kind of damaged judgment and disassociated thought process, meth users often no longer have the ability to suppress urges that could lead to dangerous and/or illegal action. Justin has been using meth for years and, although he won't admit to doing anything illegal or dangerous, his mother has a long list of his sometimes inexplicable behavior. "When he was stealing and selling things, I could understand it, he needed the money for drugs," she said. "But I can't figure out why he'd start setting fires and breaking car windows."

Further compounding the problem is the fact that the pre-frontal cortex also regulates the amygdala, parts of the midbrain that control certain emotions and memories. With no pre-frontal cortex to keep them in line, the amygdala run wild. Not only are all good feelings associated with meth, but all kinds of external stimuli—a song, a place, a smell, even a color—can bring back the idea of meth, how good it makes the user feel and how bad he or she feels without it. "The methamphetamine abuser has a pre-frontal cortex that's not doing its job of controlling the amygdala," said London. "So when the methamphetamine user is reminded of drug taking by being in a place where he or she took the drug before or even the feeling of money in the pocket that could be used to take the drug, this turns on the amygdala and other areas of the brain that are important for craving."

IT'S ALMOST UNBELIEVABLE how meth affects the brain. It's a drug that forces our brains to reward us with other-wise unattainable pleasure. Then it denies us pleasure from any other source. As if that wasn't bad enough, it also makes us forget that our actions have consequences and it constantly reminds of us of how great it is. Then it damages our brain to the point where nothing, not even more meth, can ever make us feel good again. Meth is one of those strange things that if it showed up in fiction, it'd be dismissed as too perfect to be real.

IF THIS IS REHAB,
I MIGHT BE BETTER
OFF STONED

ON THE WAY TO SEE Justin, I drove by a hipster-type guy who was wearing a T-shirt that read "rehab is for quitters." I guess he's celebrating how tough his tolerance for drinking or drug use makes him, but, from his appearance, he doesn't do much of either. A few days before, I saw a guy who, from my experience, was a more accurate advertisement for drug use. Up on the two or three blocks of Spadina Road some Torontonians ambitiously call "the Village," there was a guy standing in front of a closed pharmacy soliciting spare change. He wasn't asking for handouts, at least not audibly. He had the back of his left hand pressed tightly against his mouth for the entire fifteen or so minutes that I saw him, and held a paper cup in his right. He was tall and thin, with scabs and scars all over his face, arms and feet. His clothes were bedraggled and much too warm for the midsummer evening and his shoes were replaced by two pieces of cardboard meticulously fastened to his feet by shiny, white nylon string. I would have stopped and talked with him but I had my kids with me.

The rehab place won't let me visit Justin *in situ*, so I can only talk to him when he's not in their care. Lucky for me he's an outpatient. I offered to give him a ride home because the rehab clinic is in a city somewhat bigger than the town he lives in, but he says he doesn't like the way I drive and prefers to take the bus. He doesn't want me riding the bus with him, so we can only talk in the terminal until he is set to board.

He said that his rehab was going well, but wouldn't give too many details. I'd met him a few times, but I could tell he didn't trust me at all. He talked about his cravings, which, he said, "happen all the time." The worst, he said, occur when something—a smell, a song, even a color—reminds him of a time when he was high. When that happens, he told me, he can taste the phantom drug and even sometimes gets the shakes, along with an extremely powerful craving for meth. "It's like you're taking meth again," he said. "Except for the high." As his bus begins to board, he levels with me on one more personal note. He's learning to read again. Nothing special, just picture books with single-syllable words, but he recognizes it as a start and it gives him a sense of pride. He shows me a book that he's almost finished. I recognize it—Dr. Seuss's *Hop on Pop*.

As he said, it's a start.

WHEN I STARTED WRITING this book, I tried to find as many voices as possible. I set out a wide net for opinions on rehab and many of the more credible ones came back with the same answer—I should talk to Richard Rawson at the University of California-Los Angeles (UCLA). Carlton K. Erickson, the highly esteemed addiction research scientist from the University of Texas put it best when describing UCLA's reputation: "That is the only place where they are treating meth abusers with any degree of success."

Rawson, who earned his Ph.D. from the University of Vermont in 1974, has been at UCLA for more than two decades and is in charge of programs "ranging from brain imaging studies to numerous clinical trials on pharmacological and psychosocial addiction treatments." He is, according to his peers, the person who knows more about meth addiction and rehab than anyone else. His expertise is not limited to academics or North America. In association with the U.S. State Department and the United Nations Office of Drugs and Crime, Rawson and his team have worked in Mexico, Thailand, Egypt, Israel and Palestine. And, perhaps foreshadowing his career as a person who has found success with what others consider hopeless cases, he's a life-long Boston Red Sox fan.

Rawson has devoted much of his career to shutting down the idea that meth dependence is untreatable. It's a dangerous supposition, he asserts, because it dissuades governments and charities from spending money on meth-addiction rehabilitation. The thinking, he fears, is that if the success rate is so low, why invest? That belief may have evolved naturally because many of the places in the U.S. and Canada that were forced to treat meth addiction had never been exposed to drugs more exotic than alcohol or marijuana before and simply didn't know what to do when meth arrived. "These rural areas had not been very affected by cocaine or heroin so when they had to start dealing with meth users they had no idea what to do with them," said Rawson. "Patients were coming in psychotic, so you started hearing these horror stories that meth was untreatable. For those of us who've been dealing with heroin and crack users, it was more manageable."

Meth addiction is viewed by many clinicians the same way as trauma. "When you think of treatment of drugs like methamphetamine, you have to think of it like fixing a broken leg—treatment provides a structure to allow their brain chemistry to return to normal," said Rawson. "Their brain is out of tune, it's not working very well, and it takes a while to recover." The first step in helping a meth user kick is to bring down the psychosis. Clinicians report that the majority of people who have used meth long enough to realize he or she needs help to kick it have suffered from psychotic episodes. According to a study published in the *American Journal of Psychiatry*: "The severity of psychiatric symptoms was significantly correlated with the duration of methamphetamine use; although psychotic symptoms have been documented in users who have used methamphetamine for as little as three months and in users as young as seventeen." Other studies of equal merit have shown that casual methamphetamine users and even first-time users can suffer from psychosis. "In a study of eighty-six methamphetamine users, fifty-two had previous or persistent episodes of methamphetamine psychosis," said Rawson. "Although no other psychiatric disorder was diagnosed in the absence of methamphetamine use." So meth use actually creates the problem, rather than making an existing one worse.

While many meth users can put the psychosis behind them if they manage to give up the drug, not all of them can. "In a study of methamphetamine psychosis among 104 Japanese patients, symptoms disappeared in fifty-four patients within a week after methamphetamine abstinence and antipsychotic medication," said Rawson, "but persisted for more than three months in seventeen patients." Worse yet, even those who record no spontaneous psychosis can still suffer paranoia and hallucinations in response to periods of extreme stress long after they're given up meth.

Since psychosis is so common in meth users, common practice in hospital emergency rooms is to treat all suspected meth-related cases with antipsychotic drugs "to help calm the individual and prevent them from injuring themselves or others until the psychosis-inducing effects of methamphetamine have dissipated," said Rawson. And, as one emergency department nurse told me, "expect them to be violent."

With the patient calmed and unlikely to hurt him- or herself or others, the staff then wait until the meth has metabolized through the patient's system. Unfortunately, that can take weeks and there is a very strong impulse to take meth again to relieve the, among other things, lethargy, anhedonia and suicidal thoughts. Unfortunately, there are no drugs that will alleviate the symptoms of meth withdrawal. Rawson suggests "rest, exercise and a healthy diet."

Because meth is often used in conjunction with other drugs and its use can actually be related to other physical, mental or emotional problems, doctors generally interview meth patients about a number of issues including personal history, family history and the use of other drugs and alcohol. Cues taken from these interviews and indicators of cultural and socio-economic factors can greatly help determine what method to apply. Clinicians frequently use two tests—the standard one from the *Diagnostic and Statistical Manual of Mental Disorders* (DSM-IV) and the more esoteric Addiction Severity Index (ASI)—to determine the amount of abuse and the level of dependence the patient has acquired. These tests are backed up by chemical tests involving the patient's urine, hair, saliva and blood.

It would be great if there was an antidote to meth, but there isn't. Right now there are no chemical treatments that will help meth users recover from what they've done to their brains. But it's not for want of trying. Clinical tests with a variety of some of the most powerful drugs known to science have produced nothing more effective than placebos. So scientists are working to develop a medicine that will do something. "The discovery of a pharmacotherapy for the treatment of methamphetamine dependence is currently a major priority," said Rawson. "As clinical observations suggest that the neurobiology of some methamphetamine-dependent individuals is so disrupted and their functioning so severely impaired, that without effective medication, successful treatment with psychological/behavioral approaches is unlikely." And the company that comes up with a chemical to help stop or reverse the effects of meth on the brain could strike gold. "In our pipeline right now, we have about ten compounds in various stages of clinical trials, most of them very early on, for methamphetamine addiction," said Timothy Condon, associate director for science policy at the National Institute on Drug Abuse (NIDA). "They're all classic medications used in other areas of medicine that we're testing as anti-methamphetamine agents."

One that has shown some potential to deal with at least part of what happens to the brain of a frequent meth user is a dopamine and phenylethylamine-raising drug called Selegiline. Relatively new to the market, having been approved by the U.S. Food and Drug Administration (FDA) in February 2006, Selegiline is a drug used to combat the symptoms of Parkinson's disease and senile dementia, both of which have similar traits to the dopamine-reducing affects of meth use. Even if it does work in that area, it does nothing to treat the effects of serotonin and norepinephrine loss. And, in an ironic twist, Selegiline is chemically similar enough to methamphetamine that a good chemist could probably figure out a way to cook it into meth.

So without an effective drug, rehab clinics generally resort to the tried and true behavioral methods they use for alcohol and other drugs. Without special considerations for meth patients, things like family involvement, interventions, group therapy and 12-step programs generally do little to alleviate the problems associated with prolonged meth use. But the more successful meth dependence treatments involve all of those things. Under Rawson's care, patients stay for four to six months and undergo at least three individual or group therapy sessions a week with constant coaching. They are taught not just about what meth can do to them (they probably already know that), but also which behaviors—like drinking alcohol—can lead to a relapse and what they can do to manage their cravings. When appropriate, family members or other loved ones can be invited in to speak and other methods, like the 12 steps, can be employed.

The biggest problem with meth rehab is keeping people there. Not only is the withdrawal a horrible experience, with the body constantly craving more meth, the incentive is there to fail, not to succeed. "Throwing the onus back at a person that they're a total failure because they tried and they didn't make it, gives you the mindset that, 'Well gee, since I'm a failure already, then why should I even bother to try again?'" said Dr. Greg Peterson, clinical director of the Fergus Falls, Minnesota-based Regional Treatment Center. "I think that's a mistaken thing."

The craving for meth during withdrawal is immense. The brain has grown so dependent upon meth's help to spur the hormones that allow positive feelings that it sends out constant messages for more meth. It's often more than a person can bear. "Relapse is not the exception. It is the rule," said Dr. Holley, the obstetrician and founder of Mothers Against Meth. "Some addicts give up after two or three relapses." Sometimes the desperation for more meth can defy ordinary bounds of logic. Ricky Dale Houchens was a Kentucky meth cook whose trailer-based lab exploded, giving him third-degree burns over forty percent of his body. After six weeks at a burn unit, he was released and a month later he was apprehended while snorting meth again. "I felt bad, like I let everyone down again," he said, describing the drug as "Lucifer himself."

A significant problem with getting over meth is that most insurance companies, who have designed their models specifically around alcohol, will only pay for thirty days of care, which simply isn't suitable for meth users. "The way a lot of insurance policies are written, and managed care companies are forced to operate because of funding constraints, they want to measure progress in what's happening today that's better than yesterday," said Jim Atkins, a former meth user who now works at the respected Hazelden Foundation in Minnesota. "When someone's in early recovery, when someone's in treatment for methamphetamine addiction, you're not going to see dramatic breakthroughs from one day to the next."

If there's one method that has shown particular success, it's been what clinicians call contingency management (CM) or what the rest of us refer to as positive reinforcement. Historically, CM has been effectively used to help people dependent on heroin, cocaine and nicotine and has, at least at Rawson's own not-for-profit Matrix Institute for Addictions, shown some success in helping patients overcome methamphetamine dependence. "Individuals who have been assigned to contingency management conditions have shown better retention in treatment, lower rates of methamphetamine use, and longer periods of sustained abstinence over the course of their treatment experience," said Rawson. "Without question, contingency management is a powerful technique that can play an extremely valuable role in improving the treatment response of methamphetamine-dependent individuals."

WHILE EVERYONE from the DEA to *Rolling Stone* magazine agree's that meth addicts have about a five or six percent chance of kicking the habit if they try rehab, Rawson says he can get ten times that rate if the addicts come to him and spend four to six months at his facility. While statistics in a field like this come frighteningly close to irrelevant because of the remarkable number of mitigating factors, they're all we have.

So, taking the best-case scenario and using what most clinicians in the field agree is the best care in the world, which your insurance won't pay for, you really only have a fifty-fifty chance of kicking.

And those numbers are only of use if you can get into a facility. Justin's mother Erin told me she had to wait eight weeks in order to get him into an affordable rehab facility.

In Nebraska, a state hit hard by meth use, there is only one rehab center that accepts pregnant women and new mothers. St. Monica's in Lincoln generally treats at least one hundred women at a time and has a waiting list of at least one hundred more. "They sit on our waiting list and white knuckle it, and try to stay sober and not use substances while they're waiting," said director Corrie Wesely. "That's when it starts costing society, because we don't have a place for the people who need help to go get help."

But that's the nature of rehab. Even if you get in, do your best and follow all the rules, it's not a guarantee; it's a process. It's like school or a job or a marriage or anything else that has to be worked at. And, again, there's a little paradox there. The rehab process is trying to help people not want meth by forcing them to do what they couldn't do without meth and not giving them any meth. Getting free of an addiction is, under any circumstances, a remarkable feat.

And it's important to think about what we mean when we define recovery from an addiction. Rawson, like most, defines a successful treatment as a patient who a year later tests negative for meth in urinalysis. Putting aside the fact that there are methods for the motivated to falsify their urinalysis and the fact that meth can be entirely washed from the system in two to four days, the clinical indication that a patient isn't taking meth a year after treatment may not indicate that he or she is completely clean of other drugs, let alone doing well. Most clinical research

OCCUPATIONAL HAZARDS

The DEA has put together a list of the dangers posed by some of the ingredients used in making meth.

Acetone/ethyl alcohol: Extremely flammable, posing a fire risk in and around the laboratory. Inhalation or ingestion of these solvents causes severe gastric irritation, narcosis, or coma.

Anhydrous ammonia: A colorless gas with a pungent, suffocating odor. Inhalation causes edema of the respiratory tract and asphyxia. Contact with vapors damages eyes and mucous membranes.

Freon: Inhalation can cause sudden cardiac arrest or severe lung damage. It is corrosive if ingested.

Hydriodic acid: A corrosive acid with vapors that are irritating to the respiratory system, eyes, and skin. If ingested, causes severe internal irritation and damage that may cause death.

Hypophosphorous acid: Extremely dangerous substitute for red phosphorus. If overheated, deadly phosphine gas is released. Poses a serious fire and explosion hazard.

Iodine crystals: Give off vapor that is irritating to respiratory system and eyes. Solid form irritates the eyes and may burn skin. If ingested, cause severe internal damage.

Lithium: Extremely caustic to all body tissues. Reacts violently with water and poses a fire or explosion hazard.

Phenylpropanolamine: Ingestion of doses greater than 75 mg causes hypertension, arrhythmia, anxiety, and dizziness. Quantities greater than 300 mg can lead to renal failure, seizures, stroke, and death.

Pseudoephedrine: Ingestion of doses greater than 240 mg causes hypertension, arrhythmia, anxiety, dizziness, and vomiting. Ingestion of doses greater than 600 mg can lead to renal failure and seizures.

Red phosphorus: May explode as a result of contact or friction. Ignites if heated above 260°C. Vapor from ignited phosphorus severely irritates the nose, throat, lungs, and eyes.

Source: DEA

indicates that the damage done to the brain by meth is permanent. According to NIDA: "Research suggests serious cognitive damage, including the impairment of ability to recall word-pictures, ability to manipulate information, ability to filter irrelevant information and ability to make decisions." Just stopping meth use does not appear to begin healing. Dr. Nora Volkow of the Brookhaven Institute in upstate New York studies brains of former meth users—using positron emission tomography, which measures dopamine activity—at the onset of total meth abstinence and again after six and fourteen months. "Low levels of dopamine transporters in methamphetamine users were associated with poorer performance on tests of memory and motor skills, which did not improve with dopamine transporters after lengthy abstinence," she said. Other sources, however, suggest that some parts of the brain may begin to heal after two years of absolute abstinence. Although the damage caused to other internal organs, sexual functionality, teeth and skin can be different stories.

That doesn't mean that meth addicts can never feel happiness or read again. It just means that they must work far harder to do so. There are a fixed number of cells in the brain—you can't grow any more than you were born with. And when some of those cells that perform a specific function are dead, those that remain in the same area just have to work harder. The difficulty of recovery is directly related to how affected the parts of the brain are. Re-entering a productive lifestyle for an abstaining meth user can be as difficult as learning to walk again after a traumatic accident.

No matter how much rehab can do for a meth-affected patient, there are always things that will never come back and others that will never go away. "We have to sort through what is drug-induced—which mental health issues are drug-induced, and which might be there regardless of the drug," said Atkins, who has kicked meth, maintained total abstinence, and devoted his career to helping others do the same.

"Some of those symptoms are short term. Some of them go away. Some of them don't."

JUSTIN'S NOT AT one of Rawson's centers in California. He attends a Christian rehab in southwestern Ontario. It's not uncommon for rehab and religion to be associated. Holley, who frequently attributes Satan as being responsible for addiction, said: "The only person who can talk to your addicted kid is the Holy Spirit." While she may sound like she's out on the fringe, religion is the basis and mainstay of some of the most common recovery programs. Alcoholics Anonymous was founded in Akron, Ohio, in 1935 by two deeply religious men—Bill Wilson and Dr. Bob Smith—who were both having problems staying sober. Their organization started out as "old-fashioned prayer meetings" and the founders both described it as a "Christian fellowship." Wilson and Smith both successfully gave up drinking and wrote their own experiences down in a book called *Alcoholics Anonymous*, but to avoid confusion, most adherents just call it "the Big Book."

While the book itself is considered somewhat quaint these days, one element transcended not only the book, but the organization. Wilson and Smith distilled their plan for recovery into what they called the "Twelve Steps." Of course, 12-step programs are now in use in all kinds of behavioral applications, including meth rehab. But they still show a strong link to their religious roots and stress that faith is a vital step on the road to recovery. The *Alcoholics Anonymous* version says:

1. We admitted we were powerless over alcohol—that our lives had become unmanageable.

2. Came to believe that a power greater than ourselves could restore us to sanity.
3. Made a decision to turn our will and our lives over to the care of God as we understood Him.
4. Made a searching and fearless moral inventory of ourselves.
5. Admitted to God, to ourselves, and to another human being the exact nature of our wrongs.
6. Were entirely ready to have God remove all these defects of character.
7. Humbly asked Him to remove our shortcomings.
8. Made a list of all persons we had harmed, and became willing to make amends to them all.
9. Made direct amends to such people wherever possible, except when to do so would injure them or others.
10. Continued to take personal inventory and when we were wrong promptly admitted it.
11. Sought through prayer and meditation to improve our conscious contact with God, as we understood Him, praying only for knowledge of His will for us and the power to carry that out.
12. Having had a spiritual awakening as the result of these steps, we tried to carry this message to alcoholics, and to practice these principles in all our affairs.

Their version makes it very clear that belief in God is essential for the program to work. Not surprisingly, many other practitioners of 12-step programs have replaced the word "God" with "a higher power" for reasons of inclusion. They argue that agnostics and even atheists can be helped as long as they submit their will to the seemingly nebulous concept of a higher power. Critics counter that 12-step programs are just religious brainwashing and that their authoritarian nature takes advantage of people in need of help. They were even parodied on *South Park* in an episode called "Bloody Mary." In it, a character is arrested for drunk driving and is publicly humiliated and reviled until he enters a 12-step program. There he learns that addiction is a disease and not a choice and the only cure is faith in God. While waiting for a miracle, he becomes increasingly enfeebled and is near death when events change his mind and his life returns to normal.

But there are no vagaries about a "higher power" where Justin's going. His rehab center is funded and run by very devout Christians who work very hard to convince Justin that his only way out of meth is to (as he recites it) "form a close personal relationship with our Lord and Savior, Jesus Christ."

Although nominally a Christian, Justin didn't care much for religion and stopped going to church as soon as his mother let him. But for the sake of the rehab, he's talking the talk and walking the walk. "They tell us about Jesus and how much He loves us," he told me. "And how, if we believe in Him, we won't need meth anymore. I pray and everything but it still sucks."

COLLATERAL DAMAGE

RICHARD NORONHA couldn't believe what he was hearing. It was good news, but it made him nervous all the same. It was Daniel, his younger brother, calling, and he wanted money. Normally, Richard wouldn't even listen to his brother's pleading. After all, Daniel was an admitted crystal meth addict and petty thief. Richard knew that he had stolen from pretty well everyone he knew, including his mother, and had used all his charm and persuasiveness to cadge money from his friends and family. "Mom always wants to believe him," said Richard. "He'd say he'd have a job, but that he hadn't been paid yet, so he needed a few bucks for the subway and for lunch. She never said no."

But this was different; it wasn't just for Daniel, it was also for Sabrina, his daughter. Richard sincerely loved Sabrina and felt that she really needed and deserved a lift. Born to two crystal meth-addicted parents, she had been dealt a bad hand from the start. Her mother, Elizabeth, was in her forties at the time and had been using crystal meth for years. When Daniel told Robert that she was pregnant, Robert was immediately worried and asked his brother if he thought it was a good idea for an addict to have a baby. Daniel assured him that Elizabeth had cut down and that the doctor they'd visited actually told her that since withdrawal was more dangerous for the baby than the addiction, he recommended that she keep taking it.

Robert didn't believe him, of course, but there wasn't much he could do.

When his brother called him to tell him Elizabeth was in labor, Robert rushed to the hospital. He took the obstetrician aside and asked her if she knew that the mother was a crystal meth addict. He wasn't surprised but he was disappointed that Daniel hadn't shared that vital information with the doctors. Just as his niece was being born, Robert made the "toughest decision" and called the Catholic Children's Aid Society (CCAS).

As soon as she was born, the doctors could tell that Sabrina was suffering from withdrawal. When she was well enough to leave the hospital, the CCAS took custody. But the family "couldn't bear the thought of her growing up in a stranger's home," and Richard and Daniel's mother convinced the CCAS to let her take Sabrina. Although she became quite taken with the little girl, Sabrina's grandmother was still working and did not have the time and resources to devote to a baby, especially one suffering through crystal meth withdrawal. In stepped one of the boys' aunts who was not working, but who was so immediately fond of the girl she named a room in her family's banquet hall "Sabrina's Place" in her honor.

But it wasn't always easy. Besides the usual health problems babies face, Sabrina suffered from other ailments, including cysts on her liver and vaginal bleeding. But she was coming along and was well-loved and everyone in her family made a point of visiting her frequently.

Everyone, that is, except her father. And that is why Robert listened when Daniel begged him for money over the phone.

Daniel sounded even more desperate than usual. He had a plan, he said. He wanted to go to rehab so that he could be a real father for Sabrina. He wanted to check into rehab and get clean as a first birthday present for his daughter. Robert, who'd put up with years of his brother's begging and lies, couldn't help but relent. Sabrina deserved a father and at least Daniel was admitting he had a problem and was trying to get better. Robert didn't want to believe that his brother would never get better, so he asked him for more details.

The rehab center was in the Bloor and Spadina area of downtown Toronto, a short drive from the East End neighborhood where Daniel and Elizabeth lived. Robert drove his brother to the facility, signed him in, paid the entire four-thousand dollars fee and left. Later the same day, Elizabeth walked the six miles from where she lived to the rehab center and, according to Robert, "coaxed Daniel out." He missed the birthday, he missed the christening and, as far as the family knows, has not seen his daughter since the day she was born.

The Noronhas don't exactly fit the stereotype of the Jerry Springer-style poor, white, undereducated family torn apart by crystal meth. Richard and Daniel's father was from India and their mother from the Philippines. They decided to emigrate to Canada because most of her eleven siblings had settled in the Toronto area while his were spread around the world. They're still together almost forty years later and live in a quiet Toronto neighborhood.

Things were pretty good. The kids (the boys also have a sister) went to Catholic schools and got along well in their studies and in their neighborhood. But when marital problems with their parents emerged, it put a strange new stress on the kids, who were now in high school. Daniel, in particular, began to change his behavior. The parents stuck together in large part because they believed that it was good for the children. As

Robert pointed out, they both believed it "was better to have a troubled child in a good environment than a good child in a troubled environment."

But troubled kids seem to have a knack of finding other troubled kids, no matter what the neighborhood. Pretty soon, Daniel started hanging around with a different set of friends. "They weren't thugs or anything," said Robert. "Just kids with no ambition and no direction." And Daniel quickly became one of them. "He became disengaged from his academics, his old friends and his family," said Robert. "He and his new friends started cutting class and spending their afternoons in the ravine drinking beer and smoking cigarettes."

He eventually left high school and, through family connections, got a job in a call center for a life insurance agency but continued to live at his parents' house. After work, he spent many of his evenings at a local bar where he joined a darts league. The guys he was hanging out with were different. While Daniel was barely in his twenties, these guys were all in their middle thirties and had been selling real estate in a very *Glengarry Glen Ross* kind of way for years. They were tough guys, they worked hard and cooled off with drinks, darts, cocaine, crack and crystal meth.

Robert started receiving voice mail messages at four in the morning and wondered why. It started to make sense when a friend approached him and told him that Daniel was taking crystal meth. Robert was shocked. He knew Daniel sometimes ran around with a tough crowd, but he was an adult now and this was serious. Robert recruited his oldest cousin, a wise and strong man they both admired, and confronted his little brother. Daniel, persuasive and confident, denied the charges and Richard had little choice but to believe him.

He faith was shaken considerably when he found out that his mother frequently noticed cash missing from her purse and that his dad would sometimes wake up to find no money left in his pants pockets. Then things got really serious. One of the hardcase salesmen Daniel hung out with, Bernie, hit rock bottom. His drug use had begun to affect his performance as a salesman and he lost not only his job, but also his house. His crystal meth-addicted wife, Elizabeth, left him and hooked up with Daniel, twenty years her junior. She quickly moved into the furnished basement Daniel occupied in his parents' house. Soon the Noronhas noticed that things, ranging from a brand-new DVD player to pocket change, were missing. Still Daniel denied he was taking crystal meth. He admitted that Elizabeth had a problem, but said that's why he invited her in—he loved her and he wanted to help her. When his parents' bank accounts had been cleared out and they started getting letters reporting bad checks they hadn't written, Daniel and Elizabeth moved out.

They immediately went on welfare, but couldn't make ends meet. Daniel's dad paid their rent and his mom showed up every once in a while to fill their otherwise empty fridge. That's when they found out Elizabeth was pregnant.

Sabrina's almost two now and Daniel has yet to see her. Elizabeth drops by once a month or so, but the aunt who has her is fighting to adopt her. Daniel and Elizabeth still manage to live in their apartment as staving off eviction for long periods is relatively easy in Toronto, but have no phone and refuse to answer the door. Robert doesn't hear from his brother as much as he hears about him. Old friends still call him, livid, and scream about how Daniel has been trying to cash checks on their accounts. He also heard from American Express, wondering why he hadn't made any payments on his line of credit. Robert hadn't taken out an account with the firm, but he knew who had. Daniel had intercepted an offer from Robert's mail and, since he knew all of his brother's information, managed to open a $35,000 account in his name.

Although he thought about it, Robert didn't have much choice. He called the police. Daniel was arrested, but released under his own recognizance. As of the time I'm writing this, Robert is waiting to find out what will happen to his brother. He's tried to call, but the phone's been disconnected.

OKAY, THERE ARE lots of crystal meth stories worse than the Noronhas'. We've all heard about this or that horrible crime committed while on the demon drug. Dianne Feinstein, the senator from California who has vociferously fought against meth, has often repeated a story about a New Mexico father who, high on the drug, was arguing with his fourteen-year-old son in their car. Eventually, he pulled over, beheaded the boy and threw the severed head at a passing car. While nobody is going to say that meth use is a slippery slope on the way to beheading, it clearly played a part in this case, which (after much research) I have determined actually happened. Look at it this way: if I had a few glasses of cabernet sauvignon and ran over your cat, I wouldn't be a sadist, I'd be a drunk driver and, if you judge by the penalties we dish out, that's far worse.

I have talked with officers who actually weep when they tell me about how they have busted what they call a "Beavis and Butt-head" lab in some ramshackle hovel in some nothing town and that the six-year-old kid who had to live there asked them to take her with them. Imagine living with parents who spent their entire lives making and taking drugs. Imagine seeing a squad of men in black armor and gas masks carrying assault rifles and breaking down your door. Now imagine watching those same men handcuffing your parents and leading them, screaming and fighting, into a police car. Now imagine how much you would have had to have suffered to have decided that appealing to these invaders in Kevlar for a home is better than being sent back to your parents.

But Daniel isn't dead and hasn't killed anyone. Sure, he's abandoned his child—as his brother's said, "he's chosen crystal meth over his daughter"—but she's in a loving and stable home now. Daniel's not here for shock value. He's here because he's typical.

It often seems to be the children of users who suffer the worst for their parents' addiction. Every cop I've talked with has a story about how reckless parents endanger their kids, often by forcing them to live in close quarters with highly explosive meth labs and the poisonous and corrosive chemicals they require. Bongs full of meth residue have been frequently found on the same shelves as sippy cups (which they closely resemble) and other childhood essentials, often within reach of the children themselves. "I've seen a hot plate cooking [meth] on the floor and a toddler crawling on the same floor," said Virginia State Police special agent Mike Baker. "These children depend on you for their lives, and they're being neglected for the sake of your drug habit." In March 2006, a team from the Royal Canadian Mounted Police (RCMP) in Surrey, B.C., raided a suspected meth cook and found firearms, explosives, a marijuana growing operation and a fully stocked meth lab. In the same house, they found "a baby room with a crib, swinging chair, baby clothes and diapers." Although three men and a woman arrived at the house while the cops were there and were promptly taken into custody, the baby was never found or identified.

Labs are routinely boobytrapped with explosives to prevent invasion by law enforcement. But the chemicals themselves—as we have seen—are so volatile that the risk of accidental explosion is extremely high. Not to mention the obvious: curious children left on their own are enchanted by "strange" liquids in easily accessible bottles. And cooks and meth addicts tend to be fairly indifferent when it comes to monitoring children.

Perhaps worse than the risk, of explosion and poisoning are the cumulative effects of negligence. Doctors have repeatedly told me that a part of the brain damaged by frequent meth use is associated with impulses we might call the nurturing or the protective intuition: the positive feelings aroused when a person takes care of their children. Without a brain capable of telling you to teach, nourish and protect your children, it just sort of slips your mind. Children's welfare takes a backseat to the drug. "It's impossible to overstate the hold it has—crack's like baby food compared to meth," said Lynn Eul, an investigator from the Snohomish County, Washington, district attorney's office and a former meth user. "It addicts folks, on average, the third time they use it and permanently hijacks their judgment. They don't sleep for weeks, they defecate on the floor and let their kids starve and go naked."

"The parents' focus is on meth, not on the children," said Kathy Baumgarner, director of Child Protective Services for Smyth County, Virginia. "It just robs children of the parents they deserve to have." Although there has been an overall decline in the number of children who require foster care in the U.S., the number of children coming from meth-addicted homes continues to rise. "I think meth is a scourge and a cancer, particularly in our rural areas right now," said Tennessee governor Phil Bredesen. "I see it most acutely in the several hundred children last year that were coming into state custody because they are part of meth households. This is terrible stuff."

It doesn't always start out that way. Cheryl Barnett of Pittsburg, California, tried meth when she found that the struggles of being a single mother were just a bit more than she could handle. At first, she loved it. She found that she had more energy and more motivation than ever before. She worked harder and her house was cleaner than it had ever been. But then, meth started taking over. "There gets to be a point where you can't function without it—any little excuse and you need to have it," she said. "Pretty soon, to go shopping you need to get high, just for that energy." And, in that ironic way meth has, it eventually started to rob her of the very things she depended upon it for. "In the end, I wasn't working; I was barely maintaining the household," she said. "My children were hungry and dirty—that's when they were removed from me." Well, it's not entirely true that her children were taken away because they were thin and filthy. Acting on a tip from a neighbor, police found a small meth production lab in Barnett's home and took her kids away. Only after a long and meth-free jail term did the state consider her fit enough to return her children.

And often, the child in question doesn't even have to be born for meth to start causing it trouble. Dr. Holley estimates that about 10 percent of her patients are addicted to meth. One, she said, showed up "high as a kite. Comes in dilated nine centimeters. She is pushing out her baby. I am trying to get the clothes off this woman so I can deliver this baby and a gun falls out of her bra." Strange as it may seem in an era in which an expectant mother would be scared to take a single puff of a cigarette or a sip of coffee in public, many pregnant women still take meth. "For some the addiction is just too tough to face, they probably think that hurting the baby more by putting it through withdrawal," said an obstetrician I spoke with. "But really they're just deferring the withdrawal until after the baby is born—it will be addicted to meth and will no longer be getting a supply through the mother's body." Others aren't quite so conflicted. "Some, especially the younger ones, have even told me that the whole anti-meth message is just hype, and that they'll take their chances," she said. "Or they think they'll be one of the lucky ones."

And the mother doesn't have to be a hopeless addict to harm her baby with meth. Experiments conducted at the University of

Toronto indicate that even one casual hit can be dangerous. "We've known for a while that meth abuse during pregnancy is associated with low birth weight, cleft palates and other malformations, but this is the first research demonstrating that even a single exposure can cause long-term damage," said Peter Wells, a professor at the university's Department of Pharmacy and Pharmacology. "It's pretty remarkable that a single low dose can have such an effect." The researchers believe that the fetus can be seriously affected by even just a tiny dose, right from conception and often before the mother knows she's pregnant.

If this spate of "crank babies" seems reminiscent of the crack babies that caused a furor a generation ago, it's because the drugs are similarly addictive and have many of the same effects on unborn children. Under normal circumstances, a woman in California can expect a one in twenty chance of her child suffering from a birth defect, according to Dr. Michael Sherman, chief of Neonatology for the University of California Davis Medical Center. But, he said, that proportion quadruples if the mother used cocaine during pregnancy and increases sixfold if the mother used meth.

There can be "effects on the brain and spinal cord, such as spina bifida, effects on the heart, effects on the kidneys, where you may have water or malformation of the kidney, particularly. There is a high occurrence of problems with the development of the intestines," said Dr. Sherman. "There might be skeletal abnormalities, where they might have club foot, or developmental abnormalities or missing parts of their arms or legs as a consequence of this abuse."

One particularly disturbing side effect of meth use during pregnancy is gastroschisis, a condition in which the baby is born with some or all of his or her intestines protruding through the abdomen. While rare under normal circumstances, it shows up repeatedly when the mother has used stimulant drugs. "All of the intestines are outside the body," said Dr. Sherman referring to a tiny patient of his. "This is a common birth defect in mothers who abuse methamphetamine and cocaine before birth—particularly methamphetamine."

If Dr. Sherman's estimates are correct, about six of twenty meth-using mothers can expect their child to have a serious birth defect. That leaves about 70 percent of births involving meth that don't have those problems. But most of the remainder will have other, less obvious problems related with the drug that may not emerge until later. "The long-term consequences of its effects in the development of the brain may last for years and years and years," said Dr. Sherman. "The babies may often have sleep disturbances because it does affect transmitters in the brain. So these babies have been described as occasionally irritable babies." Deprived of stimulants for the first time, the infants suffer withdrawal much as an adult would. "Infants born to mothers who abuse stimulants such as cocaine and methamphetamine may appear lethargic and unresponsive during the first few days following birth," according to Howard Kropenske, director of the Child Welfare Information Gateway, an information outlet for the U.S. Department of Health and Human Services. "When such infants are alert, however, they are often easily overstimulated and may progress from being asleep to a state of loud crying within seconds. As they become older, infants who were lethargic during the immediate postnatal period often become more irritable and difficult to console." Under normal circumstances, these symptoms disappear around the time the child turns two. Babies born with stimulant addictions recover more quickly than adults in analogous situations because of their accelerated physical development—they literally outgrow it. And child-advocacy organizations such as Harlem's Hale House have shown that under proper care, babies born addicted to stimulants generally become ordinary toddlers and children. I don't think it's too pessimistic to think that the likelihood of a child, especially one who is extremely difficult to handle for its first two years, getting appropriate care from parents who used meth during pregnancy is far from assured. Often, children in such cases are raised by the grandparents, other relatives (as in Sabrina's case), the state or charitable organizations such as Hale House.

There are, however, a number of doctors and other professionals who deny the existence of "crack babies" and the new generation of what are now called "crank babies" or "ice babies," saying that the concept was overblown in the 1980s as a tool for American conservatives to forge support for the War on Drugs. Some studies have even shown that many of the problems associated with mothers who used crack have elevated rates among the same populations susceptible to crack use. But no doctor I spoke with was anything less than vehement in his or her opposition to stimulant use—especially meth—by pregnant women. And from what I've heard and read, it would seem that the opposition to the concept of "crack babies" is more political than scientific. Many believe that widespread acceptance and use of such terms could lead to a stigmatization of this part of the population, adding one more trouble to those they were born with. Since all symptoms can eventually disappear, there's little to be gained by labeling a normal functioning child a former "crank baby" because of the circumstances of his or her gestation.

Certainly, Robert Noronha and his family wouldn't deny that Sabrina's ongoing problems were caused by her mother's use of meth. "She was clearly in withdrawal," he said. But she, with the appropriate care given by relatives, is making progress.

While it would appear that the effects of meth are diminishing from Sabrina's life, her uncle is still having problems. Not only is his case over the American Express line of credit pending, but Robert still hears from friends and relatives whom

Daniel has stolen from or at least tried to. Again, the Noronha case is typical and illustrative of how meth can affect families and communities. Traditionally, one of the most reliable factors for mapping the progress of crystal meth has been to track the rise in crimes associated with it. And one of the best indicators traditionally has been car theft. Stealing cars isn't actually all that hard, my sources on both sides of law enforcement tell me, but what keeps most thieves away from them is the fear of being caught. Not only do stolen cars get reported quickly and are often found rolling, but the penalty for stealing a car can be very heavy. It is, I'm told, a job for a professional (and truth be told, there are very few of those on the streets) or the desperate. That's where drug addicts come in. While selling a stolen car is nearly impossible without some serious connections, one can provide all kinds of resources that can be exchanged for quick, if small, rewards. Most cars have stereos and CDs, and many, when rifled through, can produce such desired booty as cameras, camcorders, DVD players, hardware, gifts and even tollbooth change. And stealing a car to someone high on crystal meth, feeling confident, secure and nearly invincible, can seem like a lot of fun and a convenient place to snort, light up or inject again. Just as often, police tell me, the stolen car is used to transport the thieves on their way to commit other crimes.

When crack was running at epidemic levels in the 1980s, old, mostly black inner cities like Baltimore and Philadelphia saw an explosion in car theft rates. But nowhere saw it worse than Newark, New Jersey, which was once referred to as "the crime capital of the Northeast" on the TV show *Friends*. I worked at the newspaper there for nine months in the early 1990s and I can tell you that the stories you may have heard are no exaggeration. I knew two people (including my boss) who had their cars stolen from around our offices. But times change. A lot of cars still get stolen in Newark, which remains a very tough town.

But now, according to many sources, the capital of car theft in the U.S. has shifted westward, to Phoenix, where 25,651 vehicles were stolen in 2004. The chance of getting your car stolen there is about 305 percent higher than the rest of the country, according to the FBI. And it also just happens to be generally considered the American city second-hardest hit by crystal meth. While that may seem bad, Phoenix's stolen vehicle rate is about half that of Regina's. There is one vehicle stolen for every sixty-seven men, women and children in the biggest city in Saskatchewan every year. And as awful as that sounds, Regina is No. 2 in Canada.

Surrey is the second most populated city in British Columbia, but is virtually unknown outside the immediate Vancouver area. Although I'm sure the chamber of commerce would like the city to be better known as the home of Simon Fraser University or for its 5400 acres of parks, those who are familiar with Surrey know it as the white trash capital of B.C. The poor cousin to Vancouver's other suburbs, with crime rates to match. In fact, I've even heard the name used as an insult, as in "look at what she's wearing, it's so Surrey" while I was on the west coast. While all of B.C. was suffering a wave of crystal meth use, Surrey seemed to suffer worse than the rest of the area.

And now Surrey can claim the rather dubious title of car theft capital of North America, with a stunning 1700 thefts per 100,000 residents. It got so bad that mayor Doug McCallum actually stood at a busy intersection at rush hour offering free Club-style steering wheel locks to anyone who would support his plan to send local car thieves to a work camp in a nearby forest after their second conviction.

Cooler heads prevailed. Police forces from all over the Vancouver area formed the Integrated Municipal Provincial Auto Crime Team (IMPACT) and came up with a plan. Since cars were such an irresistible target, the team at IMPACT decided to use them as bait. A few late-model cars—they don't like to say which kinds—were specially rigged with video cameras hidden inside, a GPS tracking device and a computer that would allow remote access to the ignition, door locks and other controls. If the car was stolen, the police could watch it on video, track the car's location, shut it off if the thief tries to escape with it and even lock him or her in the car until officers could arrive.

Initially, some members of the team were worried that the project—like many sting operations—could be considered entrapment. But since there was no inducement to steal the car (or from it) other than its availability, there was little chance that a thief could convince a judge that the police forced him to steal. Although sometimes police will make the bait car a little harder to resist by leaving an open bag of potato chips inside. The plan has been so successful that it has since spread to areas with a high incidence of meth use including Minnesota, Texas, Oklahoma, Tennessee, Indiana, Virginia, Washington and particularly California's Central Valley where the drug originally became popular.

In an effort to raise the public's awareness of the program, IMPACT has put some of the videos on the Internet at baitcar.com. The response has been huge as the videos are frequently watched, downloaded and even distributed by e-mail on forums and on broadcast sites like YouTube. Once you've seen one of the grainy, black and white videos, you'll understand why they're so popular. From a camera and microphone mounted under the dashboard on the passenger side, viewers can see and hear a theft take place. And there's more to it than just the guilty pleasure of watching somebody break the law, there's also the unfailingly dramatic moment at which the thief realizes that he or she is in a bait car and the often pathetic and frequently funny things they do afterwards. My own favorite features a guy who inexplicably and incriminatingly talks to himself as police pursue him, repeatedly moaning "oh no," cursing the bait car program and whining about how he's "going to jail." As the police inch closer, he calmly lights a cigarette and when he's finally stopped, he begs the police not to let their dog "chew" him.

There is one video, however, that is far more frightening—even the police themselves call it "chilling"—than it is entertaining. Simply called "Oncoming," it, according to IMPACT, "demonstrates unpredictable and volatile behaviour exhibited by a young man high on crystal meth, or methamphetamine, a highly addictive and destructive drug that is widely available and cheap to buy." It begins with the thief jumping into the car, throwing his slide hammer, the tool he used to break in, into the passenger seat and stomping on the gas. As the car gathers speed and with the "fasten seatbelt" chime still ringing, he pulls a large nickel-plated pistol out of his pants and pretends to shoot it out the passenger window, perfecting his cool stance with every imaginary shot. He continues to drive, rarely looking ahead and frequently taking his hands off the wheel to fiddle with his gun. He starts pounding his slide hammer on the dashboard until he sees something and suddenly stops the car. The camera keeps rolling and captures him as he parks beside a minivan, destroys the lock and steals a GameBoy from inside.

He starts rolling again and, as the Barenaked Ladies' "If I Had a Million Dollars" plays on the stereo, he stops again and approaches another minivan with his slide hammer; but when he spots a police car, he leaps into the stolen car and speeds away. As the big V8 rumbles and the suv's tires squeal around corners, the driver gets excited and starts to scream. As first, it seems like he's yelling "fuck you!" to the cops, but as the video goes on, it gets increasingly clear that he's enjoying the chase and is actually shouting "fuck yeah!" out of pure joy. As the chase goes on, he's standing up in his seat like a kid on a roller coaster shouting and cheering himself on. Suddenly, he picks up a screwdriver in his left hand and starts yelling "oncoming!" over and over again—maybe two dozen times. He grabs the slide hammer and puts one end between his legs and the other against his chest, a position which would appear to guarantee the impalement of his ribcage if a collision activated the airbag. He starts screaming "oncoming!" and "yeah!" again until his voice gets hoarse. Suddenly, he screams "Get the fuck outta my way, bitch!" Apparently, the person he was yelling at didn't hear him because, at 89 mph, he rather happily "drives over the front end" of the car, according to the IMPACT-supplied subtitles. As the engine cuts out, he finally realizes what's going on and he starts bouncing up and down in his seat chanting "bait car, bait car." Then he pounds on the horn, which sticks. He stops and exits the car, but returns for his slide hammer and screwdriver. In the video, it looks like he gets away, but the police eventually caught up with him.

According to police, he arrived in a stolen car, stole the bait car and then stole another car in an attempt to escape. In the time he was in possession of the bait car, he hit three other vehicles and broke into three others. Incriminated by the video evidence, he was convicted and sentenced to four years in prison.

What's frightening, and enlightening, about the video isn't the amount of carnage the young man caused, but how much he enjoyed it. While high on meth, he clearly considered himself indestructible. And while armed with a handgun and a two-ton stolen SUV traveling at dangerous speeds, he really didn't care what he ran into or how much danger he put others and, perhaps more notably, himself into.

I watched the video with Kyle, the meth-using landscaper and, although he was a little disturbed by what he saw, he was pretty impressed too. "That guy is wild," he told me. "Look at him driving with one hand like that! He's really having a good time." I can't disagree with him, and I ask him if that's really what it's like to be on meth. "Well, I've never been like that, I've never stolen a car, if that's what you mean," he said. "But I can kind of understand what's going on, when you're high, sometimes it's like you're playing a video game—you're totally in control and nothing bad can happen to you." I ask him about other people, can things happen to them? He laughed and said, "it never really enters your mind."

Doctors have frequently told me about the connection between meth and psychosis and violence. "A person addicted to this stuff looks and acts exactly like a paranoid schizophrenic," said Dr. Michael Abrams of Broadlawn Medical Center in Des Moines, Iowa, a rehab center which frequently treats more patients for meth than it does for alcohol or any other drug. "You cannot tell any difference." Paranoia, alienation, confidence, aggression and a feeling of invincibility are a potent combination. According to a widely accepted model established by Dr. Paul Goldstein, a professor and researcher at the University of Illinois at Chicago and a leading expert on drug trafficking and drug-related crime, there are two distinct types of drug-influenced crime—economic-compulsive violence (ECV) and psychopharmacological violence (PCV).

ECV is defined as any crime—not necessarily what most people would consider "violence"—committed by drug users or dealers in an effort to secure their drug supply or income and it can take forms such as dealers waging war over marketing space or battling over purity down to users committing crimes to get enough money to buy more drugs. That can, as we have seen, show up as a guy breaking into your minivan to grab your child's GameBoy.

None of the users I've spoken with will admit to anything worse than shoplifting, which they laugh off and refuse to give any specifics. But their families often tell very different stories.

Remeber Erin? Her son Justin has been rendered unemployable by meth, and has stolen plenty from his mother and others. "For months, as soon as I noticed something missing, I would head over to the flea market," she said. "He used to take something from my house the second my back was turned, and sell it down there." The few dollars Justin would get for Erin's possessions would immediately go into his pipe. But that avenue of income eventually dried up for him as Erin started engraving her name and phone number on any remaining items she had that were salable. After she started threatening to call the police when she saw something of hers in the flea market, vendors there became unwilling to buy from Justin. It didn't curtail his use, although she started seeing less and less of him. "I think he started working for his dealer," she told me. "I don't know for sure, because he won't tell me; but he was never around and when I did see him, I could tell he was still using."

Other users, like Daniel, are somewhat more sophisticated, using checks, credit cards and other financial tools to get cash. In a seedy cinder-block motel with hourly rates, Edmonton police busted part of an identity theft ring in December 2005. Just as they were preparing to bust down the door of room 24, two men walked out, each talking over the other with excitement. Immediately, detective Al Vonkerman, who was leading the bust, recognized the older one, a twenty-five year old who'd been in trouble with drugs before. The other one turned out to be a twenty-one-year-old computer expert. Both were high on meth.

Inside the room, police found a laptop plugged into the phone jack, stolen credit cards, printouts of identity details for hundreds of people, hand-written notebooks detailing the pair's illegal transactions and, not surprisingly, a pair of recently used meth pipes. The police couldn't have timed it better. The thieves felt a need to get high before setting up and the younger one decided that he wanted to download his favorite video game before he got down to business. "But it was a dial-up modem, so it was taking forever," said one of the officers.

Those two were just part of a much bigger ring. "I needed to feed my drug habit and make a living," one of the higher-up workers told a newspaper from jail. "That's when I began to look into using my PC." Edmonton police made public portions of their investigation of an ongoing meth-fueled identity theft ring based in the city and the details are shocking in their simplicity. Operatives, often well dressed and presentable, would "dumpster dive"—search businesses' garbage receptacles for useful information. Mining the mountains of paper in the alleys behind banks, insurance companies, car rental agencies, cellphone stores, video rental outlets and anywhere else where many transactions are made by credit card, the workers would get all the information they needed to forge new identities. "We'd get credit check information from Equifax, credit card numbers to make payments, Social Security numbers, date of birth, addresses," said one the arrested operatives. "They would make a printout, then just throw it out." If the dumpster divers were approached by security, one of them asserted, they were instructed to act like an employee who was searching for something that they had accidentally thrown out, like a day planner.

With that information, they would buy PCs, modems and high-quality printers capable of making realistic fake identification cards. They would then congregate into motel rooms (they call them "sketch pads") and use the computers in days-long meth-fueled sessions of constant larceny. They would receive online cash transfers, order checks, acquire new debit and credit cards with new personal identification numbers, take out large loans, create shell companies capable of sending out invoices and basically do whatever they could to clean out the net worth of whoever's identity they had stolen. Like many other Canadians who engage in fraud, some of those arrested in the

Edmonton ring expressed a preference for American victims because of the difficulties authorities face with cross-border investigations and extradition of evidence and suspects.

While identity fraud and other forms of meth-related theft are prevalent, especially among men, many women choose a different route. I asked an Alberta police officer about how meth has affected prostitution in his area. "Well, it's always been around—world's oldest profession, eh?—but it seems like it's exploded around here," he told me. "And if there's a common link to all of them, it's the crystal meth." In his excellent and award-winning series "The Dasen Girls" in the online magazine *New West*, journalist Hal Herring reveals the sordid world of Dick Dasen, a fine, upstanding member of the community of Flathead Valley, Montana, who just happened to be using charitable contributions to finance a self-sustaining cash-for-sex program by taking advantage of the many meth-addicted women in the area.

Dasen was a successful businessman and a born-again Christian who, among other community services, volunteered for an organization called Christian Credit Counselling (CCC). It was intended to use charitable donations to help poor people, particularly mothers, get out of debt. But in an irony that would be delicious if it wasn't so sad and predictable, Dasen actively sought out meth-addicted women because he knew he could coerce them into sex in exchange for CCC cash or checks. The plan was simple and nearly foolproof—meth addicts always need money, meth addicts will do anything (including keep their mouth shut) for that money and they'll always keep coming back.

Prosecutors in the case estimated that Dasen ran through up to $4 million of the foundation's money, not just paying the women for sex, but also reportedly giving $2000 bonuses to those clients who would recruit more women who met his standards of attractiveness. And, in the economically depressed and meth-riddled Flathead Valley, he had little problem finding willing partners. "I just really needed that money; I was struggling to pay the bills. I wanted to buy my own trailer, and have a place for my two kids, and I was messing with all that dope," said Jenna, one of what the media began to call "Dasen's Girls" and a mother who was injecting meth every day at the time she was dealing with ccc. "My give-a-shitter was broken—all our give-a-shitters were broken."

After one of the girls died in a car accident while high on meth on a trip to visit a cook to get more meth, her mother decided to put an end to Dasen's little fiefdom. She collected the stories she knew about her daughter and other girls and brought them, along with photocopies of some of Dasen's checks, to the local police. At first the police were reluctant to believe her, although they had repeatedly heard rumors about Dasen's involvement with young women. After some investigation, they caught Dasen in the act, arrested him and charged him with one misdemeanor and nine felony counts of prostitution, felony charges of promotion of prostitution, aggravated promotion of prostitution, sexual intercourse without consent and sexual abuse of children.

Although he was eligible for as much as three hundred years in prison, Dasen actually got off fairly easy. He did not profess to be a sex addict (a condition he had already sought treatment for), as many in the media expected he would. Instead, he denied that he'd done anything wrong. According to Dasen's lawyers, all of the sex between the dozens of young women and the unimpressive-looking sixty-something had been consensual and the $4 million of other people's money that had passed between them was coincidental to their relationships. As far as the underage girls he'd had sex with, photographed and filmed, well, he claimed that they were all very convincing liars who led him to believe that they were over eighteen.

At a pre-sentencing hearing, expert witness psychiatrist Dr. James Myers testified that Dasen posed no threat to his community and that there was a "low to moderate" chance he would re-offend, although he did admit that he did not have any idea about how many women were involved, how much money was misappropriated and how much damage the defendant had caused. Dasen was sentenced to twenty years in prison, but the judge suspended all but two years. And if he continues his sex addiction therapy, Dasen could serve a minimum of twenty months behind bars.

Things didn't go quite so well for Kim Neise. She met Dasen in 2003 and became one of his girls. After getting out of jail for check forgery, she was living in her car. She was twenty-three years old, and after using meth for ten years she had withered down to ninety-five pounds and was injecting every chance she got. When a friend told her about Dasen, she jumped at the chance to meet him. As arranged, she arrived at a cheap motel and was surprised to see, as she testified in court, "a lineup of girls" waiting to see him. Not only did Neise engage in a sex-for-pay relationship with Dasen, she also encouraged two girls, fifteen and sixteen, to do the same in exchange for more money.

About a year later, the strangled corpse of a Dasen girl was found in a nearby Motel 6. Despite the fact that his DNA was found underneath the body, local police have never considered Dasen a suspect in her murder. The girls saw it differently, especially Neise, who testified that Dasen told her: "That's what happens to people who threaten to go to the cops."

Soon thereafter, Neise was arrested for forging checks again and, when the Dasen story came out, charged with aggravated prostitution. Ten months after her last dose of meth, she showed up in court about double her prior weight with a "Legalize freedom" tattoo betraying her past. Not as well spoken or well represented as Dasen, she was sentenced to ten years in prison, five suspended.

Just as meth is prominent in the world of prostitution, it's virulent in its close cousin, hardcore pornography. While I realize that there's a fine artistic, as well as legal, line between having sex for money and having sex for money in front of a camera, there are definite parallels. Centered mainly in California's suburban San Fernando Valley, the porn industry has long run on libido-enhancing, inhibition-suppressing meth. In fact, meth is firmly connected with the industry that there's actually a TGP—which stands for thumbnail gallery post and is best described as a portal for free pornography used for advertising purposes—site called "teensonspeed.com." Since the site was registered by domainsbyproxy.com, a company that specializes in keeping the identities of client domain holders secret, it's impossible to find out who owns teensonspeed.com without a court order. It's too bad, I'd love to ask them why they chose that name, but I'm pretty sure they wouldn't tell me the truth.

Meth is not just commonplace in the porno industry, it's almost a requirement if you believe actress Jenna Jameson, who's frequently referred to as the "Queen of Porn." The daughter of a Las Vegas cop and his showgirl wife, Jameson (her real name is Jennifer Massoli—the Jameson refers to her favorite drink, a popular brand of Irish whiskey) lost her mother to cancer when she was three. According to her autobiography *How to Make Love Like a Porn Star: A Cautionary Tale*, Jameson had a tough childhood—at fourteen she was gang-raped and beaten—and started taking drugs and dancing in strip clubs while she was still in high school. When she was seventeen, one club refused to hire her because of her braces, so she removed them herself in the parking lot and returned to dance that afternoon. She met and moved in with a biker tattoo artist named Jack, who cheated on her, stole her money and introduced her to his uncle Preacher, another biker. Although Preacher raped her the first time they met, she got to know him and he later introduced her to meth. Jameson, whose frank and bold book was written with *New York Times* contributor Neil Strauss, does not pretend she didn't enjoy the high she got from it.

Emboldened, she did her first hardcore porn scene to get back at Jack for cheating on her. She loved the drug and rode it all the way to porn superstardom. She loved it so much that she vowed never to speak to her brother again after she caught him stealing some of her meth.

But things are different now. Jameson is married and a mother. She's kicked the meth and reconciled with her brother. She maintains that she's happy and proud of her career but rarely makes films anymore (she doesn't have to, she makes $25,000 simply for showing up at a strip joint) and looks forward to the day she can retire. Although never apologizing or asking for pity, Jameson is perhaps at her most revealing when she writes that she very much wants her own daughter to "go to college and be a doctor or something."

PCV IS, BY DEFINITION, less goal-oriented than ECV. PCV is defined as violence caused by chemical changes within the brain itself. Meth users—usually paranoid, confident, full of energy and charged with a feeling of invincibility—frequently take chances, get into fights, resist arrest and, as we have seen, run over cars and enjoy it. At least one serious scientific study has concluded that meth-addicted arrestees don't commit more violence than other offenders, but the consensus opinion among the police, users and other people I've spoken with in the communities affected by meth disagrees. "I'm not sure where those guys get their numbers from, but they should come out with us on a Saturday night," said a police sergeant I know from a Northern Ontario town. "The meth addicts are the bad ones—they'll take a swing at you, kick you or even bite you—we always treat a tweaker with extreme caution."

Often the violence erupts when a meth user winds up in a hospital emergency room. At MeritCare Hospital in Fargo, N.D., emergency room supervisor Mary Jagim has seen a marked rise in the number of meth-related cases she sees and the amount of violence she has to deal with. "The meth has really been a challenge," Jagim said. "They're very agitated. They don't want anybody touching them. They can be very violent." She finds herself calling hospital security with a depressing regularity since meth arrived in town.

And even more frequently that violence gets turned toward the person closest to the addict. "We are seeing more domestic violence that is related to methamphetamine," said Victoria Cruz, coordinator of domestic violence and sexual assaults at the New York City Gay and Lesbian Anti-Violence Project (AVP). "There is an increase related to methamphetamine use." And, in couples where meth is a factor, the violence seems to be getting worse. "What we're seeing is an increase in the nature of the violence; it's becoming more violent," said Jeannette Kossuth, a rape and sexual assault counselor at AVP. "In relationships where methamphetamine is an issue, the likelihood of violence is greater and the nature of the violence is more extreme."

IT'S PRETTY POPULAR these days to consider drug abuse a victimless crime. The reasoning is that when people take illegal drugs they are simply making a choice for themselves that others may disagree with. Advocates frequently point out that many legal drugs like alcohol and nicotine are addictive and dangerous and long-term use can affect people's personalities in negative ways. It's an almost universal opinion that either of those officially acceptable highs cause far more damage than some, like marijuana, which are illegal. To many, the decision as to what's legal and what isn't seems whimsical, almost random.

The organized crime associated with drugs, legalization advocates say, is a result of the misguided War on Drugs. The logic is that if the governments of Western nations legalized drugs, there would be no need for illegal trafficking and that the violence that organized crime brings would be ground to a halt.

I don't actually believe that, but let's set it aside for a moment anyway. Even when the organized crime and distribution networks are taken out of the equation, there's still plenty of crime and other social ills associated with meth. Meth users steal to get cash to buy more meth (and they would if it were legal). People high on or hungover from meth commit crimes, sometimes randomly, due to a number of psychopharmacological reasons, ranging from psychosis to paranoia to hallucinations. Noteworthy crimes committed by people high on meth vary from the horrifying—gangs of partiers clubbing to death seventeen newborn calves and one boy stabbing another fatally in the heart only to drag his body out of the car they were in so he could repeatedly smash his head in with a rock—to the mystifying—a man who stuffed dead coyotes into mailboxes, another who waited patiently on a highway completely nude and holding a sign reading "need sex" and a burglar who was fashioning a crude representation of male genitalia out of his own feces when he was caught.

While meth use may be the common thread in these and countless other crimes, it's impossible to say that the drug actually caused or even had any contribution to any of those crimes. But the consensus opinion among the hundreds of police, doctors, users, families, friends, dealers and others affected by meth is that, yes, of course it causes people to commit crimes. As Herring famously asked about meth: "What's the lesson of a case in which a long series of 'victimless' crimes somehow resulted in a lot of victims?"

"BETTER LIVING THROUGH CHEMICALS"

LIKE MOST PEOPLE trying to pull a fast one, I'm looking for the weakest link. I walk up and down the front of Loblaws Forest Hill Market, a somewhat upscale grocery store, checking out the cashiers. The guides on the Internet say to find a stupid one, but I disagree. A smart cashier is far more likely to get distracted, make mistakes and let the details slide. Stupid ones, from my experience, fixate on anything they find out of the ordinary and often require help from management when they get confused. Best to avoid them altogether. Before long, I spot my target. She's about twenty, and a recent immigrant from what I guess is Russia. She's talkative and, from my observations, prone to mistakes. Perfect. I get in line.

As every good con artist knows, the best way to hide something is to be absolutely conspicuous about everything else. I smile, and ask her *kak vas zavut?*—"what's your name?"—in Russian. She grins, blushes a little and points at her nametag. Then she tells me she's not Russian, but actually Ukrainian, although most people from her country speak Russian as well because they were forced to take it in school. Okay, fine, so I start talking about Ukraine. I impress her a bit by telling her what I know about the national symbol of the three teeth, about their soccer team, and when I try out the one Ukrainian swearword I know, she laughs. It's not going to make her day or anything, but she is pretty pleased to have someone pay attention to her, rather than complain that she got the wrong code on the avocados or that she put the ice cream on top of the tomatoes.

She's happy, talkative and seems to be a pretty nice person, which is probably why she didn't notice what I was buying. As we chatted about music and art and things like that, she passed ten boxes of decongestant, two bottles of iodine, three boxes of wooden matches and three containers of lye through her scanner. She bagged my odd order; I paid cash and was off to my next stop.

Canadian Tire is an overgrown hardware store that now includes departments for home improvements, sporting goods and all kinds of other things. You can find almost anything there. So I start looking and find everything I need. I didn't have to dig for long, and hit pay dirt in the paint aisle, where I started putting a bunch of big white plastic jugs in my cart. Denatured alcohol is $3.79 for about a liter, muriatic acid goes for $8.39 for four liters, acetone costs $6.39 for 473 ml, ammonia stickers at $2.39 for 1.8 liters and little green jugs of propane intended for barbecues cost $4.39 for a 465 gram tank. Nobody bats an eye as I wheel up to the register and talk to the cashier about her purple hair and piercings. Not only does she process and bag my order, but she wishes me "an interesting weekend."

Two stops not quite a half mile apart, less than $100 spent and I have enough to make about an ounce of meth. The street value for meth in Toronto right now is about $20 for what users call a "point"—a tenth of a gram. With 28.4 grams to an ounce, I could make 284 doses if I decided not to cut it (a very unlikely scenario, but let's go with it). Should I retail it all myself, that's $5680. Awesome! If I kept it up I could be a millionaire before long.

PSEUDOEPHEDRINE is an effective decongestant that works by mimicking the body's own defenses against a stuffed nose. Commonly called Sudafed, after a very popular cold remedy that contains the chemical, pseudoephedrine also occurs in Contac, Actifed, Claritin, Sinutab, Benylin, Zyrtec-D and many other well-known and generic cold pills. I chose Loblaws' own brand because it has just as much pseudoephedrine as the name brands and it's about half the price. Besides being a pretty good decongestant, pseudoephedrine is also the most important ingredient of methamphetamine. It's the chemical that actually gets changed into meth.

But it's not an easy process and there are lots of other chemicals involved. Iodine, of course, is a time-honored part of our lives. Not only is it an essential part of our diet—almost all table salt contains iodine to keep us from getting goiters—but it can be used to purify drinking water and, more frequently, disinfect wounds. Iodine, as a valuable part of our culture, is widely and cheaply available throughout the world. There's a catch, though. Meth recipes that require iodine can only use iodine crystals. Many governments are aware of this and have clamped down on their availability, making them available only to legitimate chemists. Still, meth makers are nothing if not resourceful. Tincture of iodine, the brown stuff we daub on cuts, is three percent of iodine dissolved in distilled water and ethanol. Take the liquid out, not a difficult task for any freelance chemist worth his or her salt, and you have iodine crystals.

The matches I'll throw away. But I'll keep the boxes. The strips along the side that you light the matches with—what those in the match industry call the "striker"—are a good source of red phosphorus. I could get the red phosphorus from road-side flares if I needed more, but they're pretty expensive, so I'm sticking with matches. Phosphorus is a chemical that is so volatile that it almost never occurs in nature in its pure form. It was actually discovered in 1669 by accident. German physicist Hennig Brand was attempting to obtain various biological salts by distilling his own urine when he discovered a white residue. After putting it to a variety of tests, he found that it glowed in the dark and burned with an astonishing brilliance.

Before long, phosphorus was being used in basically every industry that required a chemical reaction, from fertilizer to explosives to streetlights. Matches had been around in one form or another for centuries, but didn't really become effective until 1831 when French industrialist Charles Sauria marketed a new type, which used a strip of white phosphorus as a striker. Although his matches were much more effective and smelled far better than earlier attempts, the white phosphorus he used was extremely toxic and there was enough in a small package to easily kill a person. Word got around and subsequently, white phosphorus became a favorite tool for suicides and murders. There's even a well-known story of a man who discovered his wife's plan to kill him when he noticed that the steam from his beef stew was glowing. The stuff was so poisonous that people who worked with it suffered greatly. Although many problems can arise from working with white phosphorus, the most well known is "phossy jaw." When someone is exposed to the chemical for prolonged periods, it starts to react with the naturally occurring phosphorus in the jawbone. It begins with toothaches and swollen gums and results in a large abscess as the bone tissue decomposes. As the jawbone rots, it emits a disgusting odor and, if the case progresses far enough, will begin to glow in the dark. But the afflicted party usually dies from organ failure long before then.

Pushed on by the overwhelmingly pathetic London Matchgirls' Strike of 1888 and later ratified by the Berne Convention of 1906, the use of white phosphorus was banned in the manufacture of matches and replaced by red phosphorus. Not only was it far less toxic, but had become easier and cheaper to process by the start of the 20th century. White phosphorus is generally only found in weapons and certain esoteric brands of fertilizer now.

The red phosphorus is the chemical that combines with the pseudoephedrine to transform it into methamphetamine, but you can't just throw them in a jar, shake them up and hope to get crank. The other chemicals are catalysts that encourage the primary pair to combine. The most important of these is lye. The chemical, also known as caustic soda or sodium hydroxide, has a number of uses from soap making (as discussed in the film *Fight Club*) to food processing, but is best known as a drain cleaner. Drano, for example, is a mixture of lye and little shards of aluminum. When the lye reacts with the oils that have built up in the pipes, it causes a heated, bubbling reaction in which the sharp-edged aluminum pieces are swirled around, literally cutting the clog to pieces.

Lye is so quick to react because it's a very powerful base. Chemically considered to be the opposite of acids, bases are simply defined as those compounds that absorb hydronium—water with an extra hydrogen atom—ions. Acids, on the other hand, are those compounds that donate the hydrogen atoms to form hydronium in water. Not surprisingly, when combined, acids and bases usually cancel each other out—although the reactions can sometimes be quite violent.

Although acid's opposite to chemists, bases work very much the same way when they come into contact with human skin, causing terrible chemical burns. In fact, lye is so willing to react with biological matter that one of its traditional uses was to get rid of animal carcasses. In a process sometimes known as "tissue digestion," unwanted carcasses were placed in a vat full of a lye and water mixture then sealed. After a period of time determined by the amount of tissue involved and the strength of the solution, the bodies were reduced to a thin, dark brown liquid. Often, some of the larger bones survived the process, but they were invariably hollowed out and weak enough to be crumbled into powder by hand.

Denatured alcohol is ethanol (the kind of alcohol we enjoy in beverages) that is rendered undrinkable by the addition of various vile-tasting and poisonous ingredients. Since alcohol has many chemical uses—primarily as a fuel and a solvent—denatured alcohol is commonly used when ethanol is needed but a potential for abuse of potable alcohol exists. Of course, some desperate alcoholics will resort to trying denatured alcohol with predictably bad results. It's so prevalent in the U.K., where denatured alcohol is called methylated spirits, that some people refer to down-and-out alcoholics as "meths." Of course, that term is rapidly disappearing as methamphetamine becomes more popular in Britain.

Ethanol plays a key role in methamphetamine production. Cooks soak decongestant pills in denatured alcohol for a day or two to separate the pseudoephedrine from the other elements. The active ingredient is skimmed off the top of the mixture and dried for use. The remaining sludge is disposed of.

Muriatic acid is the commercial name for hydrochloric acid, the very powerful stuff that your stomach uses to digest food. Although it has hundreds of industrial uses and is an essential chemical in industries ranging from treating leather to making Jell-O, its primary retail use is as a brick and driveway cleaner. As the strongest commercially available acid, muriatic acid plays a vital role in meth making by starting reactions between the red phosphorus and the iodine.

Similarly, acetone is a useful industrial solvent prized for its very low boiling point. Best known to most people as the odd-smelling active ingredient in nail polish remover, acetone is widely available at a variety of different outlets. Its role in meth manufacture comes at the end when the meth needs to be separated from the other compounds in the mixture.

The ammonia is actually a case of my overbuying. Many of the other ingredients I purchased were necessary for one particular method of making methamphetamine, but there are plenty of others. Aside from the ammonia, my shopping trip would appear to indicate that I planned to make meth using the Red P method, which is appropriate because it's the most common recipe for the Midwest, as well as the East Coast. Named after the red phosphorus used as an activator, the Red P method is considered the easiest way to make meth, but many people have told me that the product is considered to be less pure than what some other recipes yield.

In Mexico and the western parts of the U.S. and Canada, meth is generally made by using what cooks call the Nazi method. Substituting ammonia for the red phosphorus, the Nazi method is more difficult, more dangerous and easier to detect because of its horrible stench, but the product is said to be much more potent. Some say the Nazi method got its name from the idea that it's the same recipe used by the Germans in World War ii, while others believe a perhaps apocryphal tale that for generations the recipe was handed around as photocopies of an original that was written on the letterhead of a white supremacist group.

Other methods use different ingredients with more or less the same results. In Minnesota, some cooks use gun-barrel cleaner as the reagent, making a faintly greenish meth that the locals call "grimace." It's not named after the popular McDonaldland character, who's purple, but rather after the stomach cramps that often accompany a dose. One of the even more effective, but far more difficult, methods involves using lithium. A highly unstable metal, lithium is perhaps best known as a mood-stabilizing drug, but is also commonly found in some types of batteries. The cooks disassemble the batteries and carefully remove the lithium from its anode, or negative pole. "Lith works alright, but it tastes awful," said one West Coast user I spoke with. "I'd rather have regular meth."

While every good Nazi method cook knows that household ammonia isn't strong enough to yield very much meth, not all cooks know what they're doing. As one Arizona police officer I spoke with said: "If they're not crazy, they're stupid; but the stupid ones don't last very long, so it's the crazy ones you have to look out for." One cook who was perhaps more misguided than crazy or stupid was Daniel "Steve" Zeiszler, a twenty-two-year-old who worked at a San Francisco recycling plant and lived in suburban San Mateo County. A meth user, he wanted to make his own stock and bought a book on the subject. When he read that ammonia was a key ingredient in some recipes, he recalled that he'd heard that human urine contained a great deal of the chemical and it dawned on him that he could farm his own body for ammonia. And, aware that any meth that had not metabolized by his body exited through his urine, he also thought he'd be able to recycle it.

He put his theory to the test in a cheesy South San Francisco hotel room. While he was setting up, he spilled some solvent (the police wouldn't say which, but it was most likely acetone because it didn't burn him) on his arm and forgot about it. After he had everything in place, he took a break, sat down and lit a cigarette. Not surprisingly, he saw a huge tongue of flame emerge from his arm. When some of the hotel's other guests saw him running through the hall screaming and aflame, they called 911. When the fire department came, Zeiszler admitted to them that he was cooking meth and they quickly evacuated the building. Investigators were surprised to see—alongside the usual hotplate, flasks, tubes and beakers—a few two-liter Pepsi bottles full of urine.

Even his defense attorney, William Johnston, referred to Zeiszler's plan as a "really, really silly move." Noting that his client had no prior arrests and that his plan would actually have worked if he used enough urine (perhaps thousands of gallons), Johnston tried to convince the court that Zeiszler was engaged in an educational exercise that just happened to be against the law more than he was a hardened criminal trying to get rich off meth. "He is a bright, articulate young man who was wasting his life playing around with this stuff," Johnston said at a presentencing hearing. "Anybody who would—for fun—read a chemistry text should be in school instead of sitting in San Mateo County Jail." Zeiszler was given five months in prison, minus time served, and three years probation. At the hearing, he promised the court he would enroll in college, hoping to specialize in organic chemistry.

Of course, more experienced cooks go for the hard stuff, anhydrous ammonia. Normally used as a fertilizer or an industrial refrigerant (especially in the West), anhydrous ammonia is dangerous stuff not just because of its suffocating fumes which have caused a number of deaths on farms when workers have been enclosed with a source, but also because it can cause serious chemical burns, often internally through respiration. That potency makes it ideal for use in meth making and it has since become a controlled substance, making it commercially available only to legitimate users.

Since meth cooks have been largely cut off from anhydrous ammonia, black market prices for the foul-smelling gas have been known to reach $1000 per gallon. Naturally, thefts from farms and industrial sites have increased. The U.S. government's Centers for Disease Control (CDC) has recorded 1791 meth-related incidences of anhydrous ammonia theft between January 1, 2000 and June 30, 2004 that have caused "public health consequences (i.e., morbidity, mortality, and evacuations)."

Typical of them was an incident that happened in eastern Washington state in April 2004. A group of would-be cooks broke into a factory to get at its 6100-gallon anhydrous ammonia storage tank. Unable to activate the valve properly, the thieves broke it off, accidentally releasing 1500 gallons of the poisonous, corrosive stuff into the air. The man closest to the leak suffered major burns to his midsection, but the others fled. One of the firefighters who came to his rescue suffered severe respiratory irritation due to an opening in his HazMat suit. "Several roads were closed, businesses were evacuated, and a train was delayed while company employees, a HazMat team, and local police and fire departments responded," according to the CDC. "Approximately twelve persons were evacuated for eight hours, and nearby residents were told to shelter in place." Eight other people were decontaminated at the scene.

The last ingredient I bought, a small tank of propane meant for a portable barbeque, is not, as I first thought, meant to heat the mixture. With so many explosive and flammable chemicals and fumes circulating through the process, open flames can be disastrous. Instead, most meth cooks prefer electric heat, often using a stove top or hotplate when heat is required. The propane is actually another reactive chemical used in the purification process. Many cooks will often use empty propane tanks to transport other dangerous chemicals, particularly ammonia, a practice that can have tragic results.

OF COURSE, MY shopping trip was a bit easier than what many cooks actually face. Both of the stores I visited were in downtown Toronto, where meth use (let alone its manufacture) is still fairly rare outside the gay community. And I really don't look too much like a meth cook. Things are different for a pharmacist I know who operates in southern Indiana, where meth use and manufacture are commonplace. Because of U.S. laws regulating the retail sale of products containing pseudoephedrine, he has to keep his most effective cold remedies behind the counter. He must also check the identification and record certain specific information about everyone who buys any. It's an arduous business that makes the simple sale of a $4 product into a lengthy, labor-intensive transaction. Neither pharmacist nor customer seems to enjoy the logs. "They are a pain in the ass and they cost me labor," he told me. "Costs legit users time and hassle; have had multiple complaints about it."

And, if you don't have the proper state-issue picture ID in the U.S., you don't get any relief for your stuffy nose. There's no national restriction on retail sales in Canada, but many communities and individual pharmacists have imposed them voluntarily. As a drug cop from Saskatchewan told me, pseudoephedrine restrictions can be hard on people who live far from pharmacies. "The restrictions keep many smaller stores from keeping it because it's just no longer worth it, so the only place you can get it is a pharmacy and they'll only sell you so much," he said. "That's okay if you live in the city, but what if you're Joe Farmer who's a two-and-a-half-hour drive from the drug store—that can get pretty hard in the winter, when you need it."

Although the police in his area have told him that the new regulations have reduced the amount of locally produced meth, Tom the pharmacist hasn't seen a reduction in the number of meth users in his store. "We have always logged syringe sales and that kept a lot of them away," he told me. "This new log for pseudoephedrine doesn't seem to make a hell of a lot of difference, with regards to tweaker traffic."

TWO BLOCKS WEST of the Loblaw's is a Shopper's Drug Mart, one of a large chain of multipurpose stores built around a pharmacy. Besides the 7-11, it's the only store open late around our house, so when my wife said that she needed Neo-Citran at 10 p.m., it's where I went. It's also where the neighborhood panhandlers hang out. There are usually two or three of them, not always the same people, but there are regulars. They've set up a little camp of sorts there with old milk crates to sit on. For some reason, they like to collect long sticks from a nearby ravine and you can sometimes watch them smooth and shape them with small blades. They're not really breaking any laws, but they can be intimidating, especially at night.

As I approached, one of them, an obese woman I'd never seen before, asked me for some "help." Since I didn't have any cash, I told her that if she didn't have a credit card machine, I really couldn't help her out. Then she rushed over to me in a panic, with her belly (which reached almost down to her knees) shaking dangerously from side to side. "Oh! You gotta help me, you gotta help me!" I looked at her silently, waiting for here to clarify. "You gotta buy me some cold medicine, the good stuff!" I told her I didn't think I could. "Oh, but you gotta, I been coughing all day and night," she was telling me. "It's gotten so bad, I got a hernia." I told her that I really didn't think I could buy her anything, which sent her into a frenzy, "You don't believe me? I'll show you my hernia!" She started to lift up her gigantic T-shirt, and I turned and walked into the store. "I'll show you my hernia!" I heard her call as I headed in and by then it seemed more like a threat than a ploy for sympathy.

I asked a cop I know what he thought and he laughed. "There are no obese meth addicts and there's nobody who makes meth who doesn't use meth," he said. "There's a chance she could be buying it for someone the store won't serve, but getting it a pack at a time wouldn't make much sense; and she could have just had a cold."

Despite a lack of nationwide regulation, Canadian pharmacies frequently make a habit of denying pseudoephedrine and other legal items to people they suspect of using them illegally. Ivan, a pharmacist in Hamilton, about an hour's drive from Toronto, tells me that the practice is widespread. "Some over-the-counter items can be dangerous or easily made into something dangerous, so I watch who we sell them to and how much they buy," he said. "When you deny them, they sometimes make a big fuss, screaming and yelling about how they're gonna sue, about how I'm violating their rights and how they're gonna call the cops, but I really think the last people these people want to see are the police."

The idea of self-regulation among pharmacists isn't exactly new. When I spoke with one Saskatoon store owner who'd rather not be named, he told me that he won't sell pseudoephedrine to anyone with visible tattoos. And he also said he won't sell any aerosol products to any male native Canadians. "Had that policy for more than twenty years now," he said. "Just don't want that kind of trouble."

And, as you might expect, it's a phenomenon by no means limited to Canada. Similar conditions showed up all over the U.S., but sometimes ad hoc actions in both countries needed a bit of a boost to become coordinated programs.

In 1881, a number of drug company owners formed a trade association to represent the makers and sellers of over-the-counter nonprescription medicines and dietary supplements. They called it the Proprietary Association, but changed that vague and somewhat sinister name to the Nonprescription Drug Manufacturers Association in 1889. That name lasted 110 years until 1999, when it was changed again to the more touchy-feely Consumer Healthcare Products Association (CHPA). With sixty active and 110 associate members representing pretty well every drug company that does business in the U.S. and Canada—including Bayer, Johnson & Johnson, Schering-Plough, GlaxoSmithKline, Procter & Gamble, Pfizer and Li'l Drugstore Brands—is more than just a lobby group and mouthpiece for the industry, it's also its primary self-regulator. So when Congress and the media started pointing accusing fingers at the over-the-counter cold remedy companies, CHPA went into action.

At the beginning of the millennium, Kansas was hit particularly hard by meth, both use and manufacture. So, a number of concerned citizens and retailers started the Kansas Meth Prevention Project (KMPP), a not-for-profit organization that strove not just to drive meth production from the streets but to provide resources for meth addicts. Primarily, their strategy was to educate retailers and citizens (like farmers with anhydrous ammonia tanks) about the dangers of meth and strategies for its prevention. Before long, the KMPP was bolstered by support from government agencies like the U.S. Department of Justice and the Kansas Bureau of Investigation and also by the CHPA.

The immediate success of the KMPP allowed the CHPA to godfather other meth prevention groups in Georgia, Indiana, Iowa, Maine, Michigan, Minnesota, Mississippi, Montana, New Mexico, North Carolina, Oregon, Pennsylvania, Maine, South Carolina, Tennessee, Texas, Virginia, Washington and Wyoming. Similarly, an associated trade organization in Canada, the NDMAC (formerly the Nonprescription Drug Manufacturers' Association of Canada, but now preferring the acronym) bolstered analogous groups in that country.

Collectively called MethWatch, the groups do a great deal of activist work from neighborhood watches to educating rural police departments about the new challenges they face. But to cooks and their employees, MethWatch is little more than a red, yellow and blue sticker on a window. The MethWatch logo indicates that the staff inside the store have been trained in the nuances of meth and won't sell precursor chemicals or other supplies to people who appear to be cooks. They also won't sell inordinate amounts of pseudoephedrine to anyone. It also represents a solidarity among pharmacists and the community and is, at worst, an example of the lowest-hanging fruit school of crime deferral. The reasoning being that a meth cook who sees a MethWatch sticker will avoid that store and move onto another.

"When you see their sticker, you know that they know not to sell pseudoephedrine to anyone who looks too much like a meth-head or more than a couple of boxes to anybody," said David. "But there are ways around it. I know one guy back home who'd make friends with a cashier—maybe offer her a couple of bucks a pack—and she'd sell him whatever he wanted, it's not like the pharmacist or the manager can be there 24/7."

YOU PROBABLY WOULDN'T notice Steve Preisler if you ran into him. An unimposing middle-aged guy, he's balding, but sports a wide moustache on his weathered face. He's an electroplating engineer by profession, working at a factory just outside the city of Green Bay, Wisconsin, and he returns home every evening to a very ordinary house where he plays single father to his two children.

Preisler is actually much better known as Uncle Fester. He acquired the name while earning chemistry and biology degrees at Marquette University. The story goes that he had a habit of making explosions when he was working, not unlike the *Addams Family* character of the same name played by Jackie Coogan in the old television show and Christopher Lloyd in the more recent films. But this Uncle Fester didn't cause explosions because he was a sloppy or incompetent chemist. Quite the opposite. Preisler just liked to blow things up.

He also liked drugs. In 1983, two years after he graduated, he was arrested for meth possession and sentenced to probation. When he was arrested for meth possession again the following year, he was sure that he'd get another light sentence because the amount they found on him was tiny. But the DEA, which was eager to clamp down on meth cooks at the time and knew he was a chemist, subpoenaed and produced credit card receipts that proved he had bought a great deal of ephedrine earlier that year. He was sent to Waupun Correctional Institution.

Enraged at what he thought was an unfair conviction and sentence, Preisler borrowed a friend's typewriter and wrote a manuscript he called *Secrets of Methamphetamine Manufacture*. It was hardly the first meth recipe book and, according to some, not among the best. But Preisler had the good luck to hook up with Michael Hoy, owner of Loompanics Unlimited, a Washington state-based publishing company that specialized in offbeat and politically sensitive books. After already cultivating a reputation and a large following with books about lock picking, seducing teenage girls and hand-to-hand combat, Loompanics offered Preisler, who adopted the pen name Uncle Fester, a wide audience.

The book proved very popular and went into seven printings before Hoy closed Loompanics to retail sales in January 2006 due to steadily decreasing orders. He sold the rights to a number of Loompanics titles to other imprints—including forty to Paladin Press—but Uncle Fester took over his own. A visit to his Web site reveals that Fester, like most people who claim to be repressed by the larger society around them, considers himself something of a misunderstood genius. "Since 1985, everybody's favorite Uncle has been writing the books which have defined the field of clandestine chemistry," the introduction to his online store reads. "My books have been described as the pinnacle of twentieth-century underground writing, and through them I have transformed this genre."

But Uncle Fester doesn't just write about making drugs. Besides co-authoring a book called *Bloody Brazilian Knife Fightin' Techniques*, he's written two popular books—*Silent Death* and *Home Workshop Explosives*—which instruct readers on how to make chemical weapons and bombs. When a reporter from CBS News asked him if he thought his books were of any use to terrorist, he denied it. "Maniacs generally do not have too much between the ears," he said. "They can pick up a book and they don't get past the table of contents."

When Aum Shinrikyo, a Japanese religious cult, intentionally released homemade poisonous gas in the Tokyo subway, it killed twelve people. Sarin, the gas they made and used, is a chemical that attacks the central nervous system and is lethal even in tiny doses. It was developed by German scientists in 1938 as a pesticide and stockpiled by the Nazis in World War II. They never used it on combat because they thought its horrifying effects would lead their enemies to be desperate for revenge. It was used by Iraq, however, in its long war with Iran in the 1980s and against internal insurgents not long afterwards. When investigators raided the Aum Shinrikyo compound they found a copy of Uncle Fester's *Silent Death*, which includes a chapter on the manufacture of Sarin. Not surprisingly, Uncle Fester, who describes himself as "the most dangerous man in America" and *Silent Death* as "a how-to manual of chemical warfare" admits to no connection. "I'm rather sad that that happened; but I don't feel responsibility for what they did," he said. "They're the ones who did it."

David, a former cook from Saskatchewan, has never heard of Uncle Fester. "I suppose I was aware of the fact that there are books with meth recipes out there, but they're hard to get here I think," he said. Canadian Customs officials routinely impound books, magazines, CDS, DVDS and other media that is found offensive—including instruction manuals for the enterprising "home cooks."

"I learned to cook from my cousin's friend Jim," says David, "then I forgot some of it. But he died, so I couldn't ask him and I had to sort of take what you might call a refresher course on the Internet."

It's not hard. A search on Google will turn up dozens. Many are marred with poor spelling and bad grammar—which is a touch disturbing in a process which requires such exactness—but they generally get the idea across.

The instructions might be correct, but can be hard to follow and leave plenty of room for interpretation. Unfortunately, judgment calls can easily lead to disaster; the trial-and-error method doesn't lend itself to the field of clandestine chemistry. Worse yet is the fact that there may be just as many false recipes on the Net as there are accurate ones. I showed a bunch of recipes to David, the cook who said he's quit. Some he approved, some he couldn't understand, and more than a few he said were "total bullshit." One, he told me, was potentially suicidal.

"I'm no expert or anything," he said. "But that's gonna blow you up pretty much before you can do anything about it."

The problem with getting meth recipes from the Internet is the same as with most things you can get from the Web—you have to have faith in the provider. Aside from a few people like Uncle Fester (who was outed), the authors of these recipes remain anonymous. While their reasons for wanting to hide their identities are obvious, it also limits their accountability.

Even if you follow the correct instructions to the letter, meth making is still a very dangerous business. According to one Michigan cop I spoke with, the majority of the meth-lab busts his department achieves happen after an explosion. Problems arise from a variety of sources, ranging from imprecise equipment, substituted ingredients and, from what police often say, overall incompetence. "This isn't three guys in lab coats working in a controlled environment making pharmaceuticals," said Cpl. Jason

Grellner, head of the drug task force for Missouri's Franklin County. "It's more like three guys in overalls making moonshine—and not really having any idea what they're doing." Most often, a spill or an accumulation of flammable fumes will result in an explosion and fire. They are so common that some states have passed laws that allow meth-lab fires to be tried as arson, which generally carries stiff penalties and prevents payouts from insurance covering accidental fires. "If they're cooking drugs and set something on fire, they shouldn't be able to come back later and claim it was an accident," said Ken Calvey, a Republican who represents Del City in the Oklahoma House of Representatives and an author of one such law. "It's dangerous. They should know that. They shouldn't be able to profit from criminal acts."

In a trailer outside his home in Scottsville, Kentucky, Ricky Dale Houchens and his buddies were enjoying a meth high when one of them suggested they make some more. Since Houchens was the host, he volunteered. When he noticed that one of the pyrex beakers on the hotplate was bubbling just a bit too vigorously, he decided to remove it from the flame. As he carefully lifted the container, the bottom fell out and the mixture splashed onto the hot burner. The resulting explosion seared Houchens in a storm of flame. "I felt my face just melting," he said. "The skin was running down my arm just like lard."

With third-degree burns over 40 percent of his body, Houchens was taken to the Vanderbilt University Medical Center's Regional Burn Unit in Tennessee, which handles the most severe cases in the area. Unfortunately, he arrived at a very crowded place. As Houchens was arriving, doctors had just finished treating a nineteen-year-old girl who spilled some of her mixture on a burner and caused an explosion. Molten plastic from the walls of the trailer she was using as a lab became embedded in her face and it took doctors hours to chisel them out before they could begin on reconstructive surgery. The DEA busted about 1200 meth labs in Tennessee alone in 2004, four times as many as they found in 2000. "For every lab we find," said Ed Synicky, an agent with the California Bureau of Narcotic Enforcement. "There are ten others out there we don't know about." It's hard to believe that's not true in Tennessee as well.

"What drunk drivers are to emergency rooms, meth is to a burn center," said the head of the Vanderbilt burn unit, Dr. Jeffrey Guy, pointing out not just the proportion of his patients who are there because of meth, but also how many of them lack sufficient health insurance. The bill for Houchens' visit to Vanderbilt was $553,000, but Kentucky's state-provided insurance only covered $100,000 and the hospital had to eat the rest. Since the unit is absorbing between $5 million and $10 million in unpaid care, its very existence is in doubt. "I don't know if we'll have a burn unit five to ten years from now," said Guy.

He's not being unduly alarmist. Despite thirty-three years of award-winning service and a series of campaigns to raise funds that included a voluntary checkbox on the state tax form, specialty license plates and an annual motorcycle rodeo, the Mississippi Firefighters Memorial Burn Center in Greenville, Mississippi, closed its doors for good in July 2006. Hospital officials and others indicated that the costs associated with treating huge numbers of uninsured or state-insured meth-related burn victims was just too much for the hospital to bear. People who suffer serious burns (no matter what the cause) in Mississippi must now be transported out of state for treatment, placing further stress on already overwhelmed burn units like Vanderbilt's.

But let's suppose that you possessed a good recipe, the right ingredients and proper equipment. Let's also assume that you were precise, careful and inconspicuous enough (and that's not easy when you're high, psychotic and/or paranoid as users can be) to make meth without blowing yourself up or getting caught by neighbors or the police. You still have to sell it, which creates

---

HAPPY BIRTHDAY! LETS GET HIGH

Kristina Landry of Everett, Washington, really missed her boyfriend so she sent him a home-made greeting card. And when Joseph Van Cleave, who was in Seattle's King County Jail awaiting trial on a firearms offense, received it, he was delighted. Not only was there an illustration and a poem from Landry, but the paper had been soaked in liquid methamphetamine. Van Cleave cut the card into squares and sold them to other inmates for $35 so they could chew them and get high.

Investigators recorded a telephone conversation between Van Cleave and Landry in which he indicated he had sold a square to another inmate, Corey Lamos. All three were arrested and charged with distribution of methamphetamine.

Source: KING-TV, The Associated Press

---

major problems of its own, and get rid of the mess without being detected.

Apache County is located in the Northeast corner of Arizona. It's a long strip of land about six times longer from north to south than it is east to west. It's a dry land (less than one in 800 acres has any water) with a population made up primarily of Navajos, although its most famous residents include the Udall political family. The northern half, cut deep with canyons and dominated by the Petrified Forest, is sparsely populated (and has little to do with the south, which has some excellent, if dry, pasture land).

In the fall of 1998, twenty head of cattle mysteriously died at once. Although the autopsies showed high levels of various toxicities, it was not conclusively determined what poisoned the cows. Many in the area blamed jimson weed, which does grow in the region and has flowers that can poison and kill cattle, but which blooms only in spring.

Suddenly, the reason for the dead cows became abundantly clear. Evidence collected in the case of a stolen car resulted in the bust of a huge meth lab just outside the town of Show Low. Three brothers—56, 62 and 64 years old—were arrested and thirty-nine weapons, including a Mac-10 submachine gun which had been illegally altered for fully automatic fire. The boys went down pretty easily; there wasn't a shot fired, and the case against them was pretty solid.

What alarmed the residents of Apache County, however, was how much poison had been dumped into their water, ground and air. According to researchers at the University of Arizona, each pound of meth manufactured results in six pounds of highly toxic waste. The Show Low lab was making about fifteen pounds of meth a day. A year of work—not uncommon—(not including weekends and holidays), would create 22,500 pounds of lye, muriatic acid, iodine, red phosphorus and a variety of other toxins released into the Little Colorado River. Police found 550 pounds of red phosphorus alone at the site. With tens of thousands of labs being busted every year, that puts a lot of poison in our environment.

The effects of toxic residue from meth labs has been linked to brain damage, as well as respiratory and immune system problems. The cops I spoke with really hate busting meth labs. "I would rather investigate a homicide than a meth lab," said Lieutenant Andrew Tafoya, the man in charge of the Show Low investigation. "These labs are a logistical and environmental nightmare."

Sometimes the labs have so contaminated the property on which they sit that the police cannot confiscate the property for resale. The cleanup of the Show Low lab, for instance, cost taxpayers more than $100,000.

Labs as big as Show Low are rare outside of Mexico these days. It's dawned on meth makers how little start-up cash they actually need to make the drug, and they have responded by setting up smaller and more mobile labs. The small-scale cooks, however, tend to be less scrupulous about both how much waste they create and how they dispose of it.

Among the most "impressive" might be the lab set up by Eddie Young in Kingsland, Georgia. It was security staff at a K-Mart department store who first noticed that a scruffy-looking customer was behaving oddly. The customer—later identified as Young—was entering the store's men's room after every purchase, then exiting empty-handed. He made repeated trips to the pharmacy (where he bought cold pills rich in pseudoephedrine), then the sporting goods section (where he bought tanks of propane). They called the police. The cops in the Okeefenokee region have enough experience with meth to bring meth test strips with them on every call. Big surprise, Young tested positive. So did the crystals he was carrying. It turned out Young was actually manufacturing small—but potentially profitable—amounts of meth in a K-Mart men's room.

Very few meth entrepreneurs, fortunately, have Young's audacity. More often, cooks make meth with what cops call "trunk labs," complete meth-making facilities that can fit into the trunk of a car. "The small labs contain flammable solvents, chlorinated solvents, acid bases," says Scott Logan, president of Envirosolve, a company the DEA has hired to clean up labs throughout the southwest. "We find just about every toxic food group."

What makes the trunk labs so successful—and difficult for law enforcement to track—is their mobility. Meth makers are increasingly setting up shop in obscure or remote areas—like national parks and forests. Lots of people go there, lots of traffic, but there's also privacy. Rocky Gardom, a law enforcement agent with the U.S. Forest Service, spoke about a trunk lab he busted in Apache National Forest. "They were in a little side canyon and had been cooking right next to the vehicle," he said. "They had set up tents and had everything laid out. It looked like they planned to be there a while." But their camping site looked a little different from all the others—a circle of dead trees. "We had one mobile-home lab that had been operating for several years on private land within the boundaries of the Sitgreaves National Forest," he said. "We found some large ponderosa pines that were one-hundred-and-fifty years old killed off by the fumes."

Most trunk labs, however, are set up in motel rooms. It makes perfect sense. With the help of a "Do Not Disturb" sign on the door knob, a cook can go for days without interruption. And, by leaving a cash deposit or a stolen credit card, he or she can pack up and move on without a trail to follow. Most trunk lab cooks use the Red P method, because the anhydrous ammonia used in the more traditional Nazi method reeks enough to attract curiosity and complaints from motel guests and staff. In most cases, though, what they leave behind is a potentially lethal mess that penetrates the furniture, the walls and ceilings with toxic chemical residue.

Dave Morris is a chemical engineer who runs a business cleaning up crime scenes for the Seattle police. Since 1999, he said, meth labs have accounted for "about ninety-five percent" of his business. Since the fumes accumulate in any porous material, things like bedding and furniture are disposed of immediately. "The mattresses go first." He also saws them in half to prevent any further use.

According to guidelines set out by the government of Arizona, "all porous materials such as carpet, bedding, upholstered furniture and related items will be removed and disposed of. All stained materials from the laboratory operations, including sheet rock, wood furniture, wood flooring, and tile flooring will be removed and disposed of." The cost can be staggering—especially for taxpayers who are forced to foot the bill when labs are discovered on public property. Morris charges $3000 on average to clean a motel room, and owners simply have to eat it because the government won't pay for it and neither will insurance.

Morris says business comes from the owners of rental houses and apartments, too. Meth-making tenants set up shop then—often literally—disappear overnight. Or they're arrested or injured or killed in a fire. Since decontaminating an entire house is much more expensive than treating a motel room, Morris says landlords will sometimes try to get a cut rate by trying to convince him that the tenants only ever used a shed or the basement to cook. It's a tough sell. Meth cooks spread chemical contamination wherever they go, Morris says. "Where did the cook go to weigh it up?" he tells me. "I guarantee he's going to the kitchen table. Then he'll clean up in the bathroom and drop dirty clothes in the bedroom."

Fortunately for Morris, business is booming.

IT'S NOT JUST A dirty business, it's a dangerous one. According to a study by the state of Colorado and the National Jewish Medical Research Center: "Over fifty percent of the officers involved in the investigation of clandestine methamphetamine laboratories have experienced symptoms involved with these investigations." The most commonly reported symptoms are respiratory complaints. Police have told me repeatedly that they consider busting meth labs to be the most dangerous and unpleasant part of their jobs.

David doesn't cook anymore. He did for a little while, back in Saskatchewan, but lost his desire to do so after a friend of his was badly burned in a fire.

"It gets to you after a while, the fear," he told me. "You're scared of blowing up, you're scared of getting poisoned and you're scared of getting caught." I asked him if it was harder or easier to cook when you're high.

He laughed. "It's a toss-up," he said. "You're more motivated, but you're also pretty paranoid."

The deciding factor for him was when the bikers moved into his town. Actually, there had always been bikers around and he had dealt with them before on an individual basis, but he started to see things change. "Before a guy would ask what I had," he told me. "Then later on, it was a different guy from the same club, he started telling me what I had to make for him." He also, David said, made it clear to him that he was not allowed to sell to anyone else. And that was a problem. David had a few steady customers, most were old friends and some were friends of friends and none of them wanted to have to pay inflated prices to a middle man. Most just grumbled, but a few threatened. One, a guy named Justin, told him that if he didn't sell directly to him, he would bring down the wrath of the Indian Posse, a large and much-feared gang made up primarily of native Canadians. David wasn't sure if that would ever happen—"I don't even think he was an Indian, but he could have connections; he said he had friends in Winnipeg, so you never know"—but it did make him realize how deeply he had gotten into the world of organized crime.

He fled from the prairies and, like many Canadians who want to leave home in the rear-view mirror, ended up in Toronto. There are bikers and gangs there too, but so far nobody important has recognized him as a cook and nobody has asked him for anything.

He still uses meth, but doesn't feel a need to cook it.

"When I first got to Toronto, I didn't really know too many people, so it was really hard to get any," he said. "When what I brought with me from back home ran out, I started using coke, but it wasn't the same." The guy who sold him the coke, introduced him to a guy who could get him meth. "Gianni mostly just sells X [ecstasy], but he can almost always get his hands on some meth—charges me more than double what I paid back home, though."

HOME COOKING

WHEN BRIAN introduces me to his friend James, I can't help feeling a bit disappointed.

Drug dealers always seem to look the same, no matter where you find them. James is, like they all seem to be, dressed in wildly expensive designer clothes that are garishly, almost ridiculously, mismatched. He has plenty of gold. His crucifix pendant often clangs against his Sagittarius necklace when he moves around.

He has a big Gucci watch and a big diamond ring. His head is almost clean shaven, but a light fuzz of dirty blond hair no longer than an eighth of an inch gives his scalp a little color. He's young and thin, but has deep lines in his face and bags under his piercing blue eyes. Like most drug dealers, he has lots of tattoos. Like a lot of dealers, he has neglected to fix his teeth.

Unlike users, dealers tend to be very outgoing and gregarious. James smiles and shakes my hand before Brian even acknowledges me. "You must be Jerry."

I tell him I am and we find a table where we can talk. James speaks in bursts and never seems to be at a loss for words—he never seems to inhale. He talks much faster than I can take down notes, but after every sentence he lets out a little noise that I think is supposed to indicate laughter, but doesn't seem to have any root in mirth. He's excited about being quoted in a book. He jokes that it'll be good for business.

His story is typical. He's from a small city in Eastern Ontario, got along well with both of his parents and is proud of his family's roots from Northern Ireland and Iran. Although he's very smart (he assures me), he didn't do well in school because he found it rigid and boring. He started smoking pot in eighth grade and was selling it by the tenth. He left high school before graduating because he found it boring, too, and "didn't do much but have fun" for two years until a guy he knew in Toronto offered him a job at a bar. He jumped at the chance to go to the Big City, but hated the job. Rather than bus tables, he started going back to Peterborough early in the week (bringing his laundry along for his mother to do) then returning to Toronto with clean clothes and enough weed and hash to sell at the bar and make a decent living.

"I still hung out there after I quit," he smiles. "And I even still lived with the manager, he was cool."

By his standards he was making a good living, but when he met another dealer who was making way more money selling coke, he was all ears. "He had it good, drove a Jaguar and everything," he reminisces to me. "But he wanted way too much for coke, I just didn't have that kind of money. So he asked me if I could afford to sell ecstasy—and I jumped at the chance."

Ecstasy is a drug that has a lot in common with meth. Discovered by accident by a German chemist in 1912, methylenedioxymethamphetamine (MDMA) was originally intended as a styptic, a drug to control bleeding. Experiments conducted by the U.S. Army revealed its mood-altering effects and MDMA would eventually be prescribed—mostly by New York City psychologists Alexander Shulgin and Leo Zeff—as an antidepressant in small amounts in the 1970s. Benefits reportedly included increased empathy, motivation, confidence and sex drive. It just made people happy. Naturally, people started to take the drug without a prescription and its use slowly started to spread throughout the U.S.

By the 1980s, MDMA—by then usually called ecstasy, XTC, X or E—had become a very popular recreational drug. Particularly common in the gay community, and with high school and university students, MDMA use became synonymous with the rave culture of all-night dances that were emerging at the time. Ravers were openly seen sporting pacifiers to help control the constant teeth grinding that comes along with repeated MDMA use. MDMA users started wearing baseball caps and T-shirts with big Xs on them to indicate they were selling. Finally outlawed in 1985, MDMA remains an extremely popular drug despite links to Parkinson's disease and other brain disorders.

I ask James about it, and he says he liked it a lot. It is way more expensive than weed, he explains, but cheaper than coke and easier to sell. He can get $40 for a single pill, he says, which only costs him $12 to $15 depending on how much if it was around. Frank, the guy who supplied it to him, couldn't get it all the time. X kept getting harder and harder to find for anyone in Toronto.

Unlike meth, which is easy to produce, MDMA is much more complicated and requires some high tech—and expensive— equipment and skills.

Frank had been pushing him to try meth, James explains, but he didn't want to. Like many, he associates meth use with rural white trash, something he was trying to get away from back home. But then Frank told him that the MDMA that he was selling (and taking) were actually about half meth and some were all meth. "He told me 'it's all the same thing anyway,' so I thought, 'what the hell,'" James says. "And now I don't even sell X any-more—I like it better, but it's too hard to get and costs way more."

He was selling a point of meth—a tenth of a gram—for $12, but a lack of supplies on the street and increased police attention have allowed him to up the price to $20. He still gets it all from Frank, but doesn't know where Frank gets it. I ask him if Frank was a biker.

"I don't think so," he says. "He's got short hair and he's in pretty decent shape."

Apparently the stereotype of the long-haired biker with a huge beer belly still exists.

Actually, two cops and a dealer I know assure me that Frank isn't a biker, but that he'd really like to be and has very close con-nections with a local club. That's not uncommon in Canada, where most meth distribution is handled by motorcycle gangs and their extended network of friends and employees.

"If you're doing something illegal in Canada," one Ontario cop told me, "like drugs or firearms or prostitution or whatever, the thing in your hands has almost certainly gone through a biker's hands at one time or another. They have their hands in every pie, if they were a legal corporation they'd be in trouble for having a monopoly."

While most of the Canadian cops I've spoken with have, on the record, stopped short of putting all the blame on the bikers, others are more willing to point the finger.

"They do, there's no doubt—to the extent they are financing individuals who can set up labs and make the product, and reap-ing profits from it," said Al Haslett, head of the RCMP's organized crime intelligence branch for southwestern British Columbia. Criminal Intelligence Service Canada (CISC), the government's crime analysis unit, agrees emphatically. Its 2004 annual report states that the Hells Angels derive "significant financial income from various criminal activities across the country such as prostitution, fraud and extortion. However, drug trafficking, particularly cocaine, marijuana and increasingly methamphetamine, remains the primary source of illicit income."

A police informant who infiltrated the Hells Angels clubhouse in Winnipeg, arduously gaining the trust of many members, detailed a great deal of drug trafficking by the bikers, particularly in meth. One full-patch member, known both for his erratic behavior and for trafficking meth, had befriended the informant. Suddenly one day, the dealer turned on him, accusing him of buying meth from other bikers.

"You're always talking about the crystal. Who else you been talking to?" the biker asked. The informant assured him that he was his only source for the drug. "Really?" the biker demanded. "You sure you haven't been talking to [two other bikers]? Don't you lie to me. Don't play me like a third stringer."

The informant's testimony revealed in detail how the bikers do business. He described a typical transaction as beginning with a coded text message on his cell phone. He would then drive to a local doughnut shop, with a bag containing $40,000 on the passenger seat. He would park in front of the shop and go in. As soon as he was inside, another car would pull up next to his. The driver would then take the $40,000 and replace it with a kilo of meth. The second man, he testified, was working for a full-patch Hells Angel.

Bikers themselves occasionally acknowledge how dangerous meth can be. In April 2006, when eight members of the Bandidos motorcycle gang were shot to death near Shedden, Ontario, it basically wiped the gang out of Canada. Not longer thereafter, Wayne "Weiner" Kellestine—one of the few full-patch members of the Bandidos left alive—was arrested along with four co-conspirators. Almost as soon as the investigation began, the Ontario Provincial Police (OPP) referred to the slaughter as an example of "internal house-cleaning." The scenario they presented was that the men who made decisions at the Bandidos headquarters in Texas were less than impressed with the results they were getting from their fledgling Canadian operation and sought improvement from a violent staffing overhaul. It certainly made sense, the Canadian Bandidos were basically stumblebums who couldn't turn a profit if their lives depended on it (and it apparently did). And these sorts of layoffs by execution are hardly unprecedented in the biker world—one Montreal Hells Angels chapter exterminated another in 1985 primarily because it wasn't pulling in enough profits from the drug trade. When he was informed of the OPP's theory, the man who most say was responsible for setting up the Bandidos chapter in Canada—Ed Winterhalder, former president of the Oklahoma Bandidos—shouted that it was "bullshit." He presented his own idea. "The person who did the killing must have been a meth-head," he said. "Usually they have been up for three or four days and sleep deprivation does some strange things to you."

Meth appealed to the bikers in Canada for much the same reason that it did to their American counterparts as many as forty years ago. It's a great high, it's highly addictive, it's easily concealable, *and* it can be made domestically using easily obtainable ingredients. Marijuana is grown in Canada, but to make any real money, you have to sell massive amounts. So many people grow and sell it, that there's really no way to cultivate and maintain a dependent customer base. The other major drugs—cocaine, heroin and MDMA—must be imported—most from highly organized and heavily armed criminal syndicates in foreign countries. Supplies are heavily dependent on a cartel's organizational sophistication. Not to mention confiscation: a bust anywhere along the importation route and the entire supply of "product" is off the shelf for good.

Meth production, however, is much more reliable, as long as lab explosions and police raids are kept to a minimum.

Biker-controlled labs ensure a smooth and continuous supply of product by keeping their labs small and by employing many cooks. If one cook catches fire or gets arrested, it won't have a significant effect on the overall amount of product available. According to the CISC's 2005 report, "the bulk of this methamphetamine is manufactured domestically in Canada in small clandestine laboratories, though larger operations capable of producing 4.54 kg [ten pounds] or more in one production cycle have been encountered occasionally."

In Edmonton in 2002, the owner of a warehouse hadn't been paid rent in a while. He sent letters to the renter, and made many calls, but there was never a response. Frustrated, he finally sent an employee down to the site to discuss the problem with the renter. There was nobody on site, however, but he did find chemicals, lab flasks, protective respirators and books about how to make methamphetamine. He called his boss, who promptly called the police.

If the tenants had kept up with their rent, the Edmonton police may have never known about a lab that was later labeled the "Wal-Mart of Meth." Police were impressed by the size of the operation and also its efficiency: different parts of the warehouse had been carefully screened off and dedicated to different tasks in the production process, and all the chemicals and work sites had been clearly labeled. "It's a huge lab, and for Edmonton particularly, it's a superlab," said Sgt. Pat Tracy, one of the officers who arrived at the scene. "It's like a large retail store."

The lab had only been up and running for an estimated nine days, Edmonton police estimated, but it was making a remarkable amount of drugs. Judging from the amount of chemicals found and the facilities in use, the factory could produce around fifteen to twenty pounds of meth in a four- to six-hour shift. If it was staffed around the clock, the police estimated that it could pump out more than $1 million worth of meth a day. They found seventeen pounds of completed meth at the site.

One clue, however, quickly indicated to the police that the cooks might not have been the seasoned professionals at first expected. "Investigators noted splatters on one of the walls that leads them to believe an explosion had occurred," said Annette Bidniak, the Edmonton police's information officer. "Likely caused by improperly mixing chemicals." The stockpiles of chemicals—if ignited—could "level six city blocks."

In a twisted but economically brilliant twist on a mentoring program, I learned from sources that lab bosses expect meth cooks to teach the trade to at least ten associates. Unfortunately, not every pupil proves adept at mastering the intricate chemistry of the process, and plenty blow themselves up before they graduate. Subsequently, meth cooks are prized and highly sought after by biker gangs. They may be lured into the gang by favors—the CISC once displayed a now-famous photo to police and media of a small-time meth cook partying with NHL coach Pat Burns and hockey star Ray Bourque along with charismatic former Hells Angels national president Walter Stadnick to indicate how bikers demonstrate the perks of association.

If they can't woo the cooks, they'll intimidate them.

"Yeah, the bikers will do that, they won't say exactly what they'll do, but they give you the idea that it's in your best interest to co-operate," said David, the cook from Saskatchewan who moved to Toronto when he decided to stop making meth. "Their interest in me was what made me decide that it wasn't safe to stay in Saskatchewan." And, if they can't recruit a cook, they may choose to get rid of him. There were instances in the war between the Hells Angels and a rival motorcycle gang, the Rock Machine, in the 1990s when either side would assassinate a cook who was working independently or with the other side. Jacques Ferland was a skilled cook who operated in Grondines, a suburb of Quebec City. He worked on his own and occasionally sold to the Rock Machine. But on January 29, 1995, he received two bullets in the head from Serge Quesnel, a professional assassin hired by the Hells Angels just up the St. Lawrence in Trois-Rivieres. About a year earlier, three Montreal-based Hells Angels operatives were arrested in Kingston, Ontario. Although police found two handguns (one stolen), a shotgun, ammunition for all three weapons and an ounce of hashish in the car, one of the men was allowed to go free. Under interrogation, Dany Kane and Michel Sheffer copped to everything (which was odd, considering they both had criminal records, and Denis Cournoyer didn't, and because it was his car they were riding in).

It's probably not a coincidence that Cournoyer was also one of the few skilled meth cooks in Eastern Canada at the time.

Similar situations exist in other countries where meth is enjoyed as well. "In Auckland particularly, you can't manufacture or distribute methamphetamine without the sanction of an outlaw motorcycle gang because if you do and they find out, they will come and say, 'You are now working for me,'" said Sgt. Darryl Brazier, an organized crime specialist for the police in Auckland, New Zealand, a region traditionally served by meth imports from southeast Asia but with an increasing number of local cooks. "People have been hurt quite badly because of their non-co-operation, but of course those people are not interested in making a complaint. They go to hospital and get treated for broken knees, broken legs, broken arms. That's the warning. So next thing they are manufacturing for the gangs."

The bikers themselves, I've learned, don't sell drugs as retailers. A biker will recruit a person who so desperately wants into the gang that he will (or convinces the biker he will) gladly do jail time in return for a promotion to member or even prospective member should he get caught rather than inform on his boss. In turn, this wannabe finds street-level dealers that he feels he can trust. Both the biker and his direct underling handle the drug as little and as discreetly as possible and always use "obscuring" methods to foil police, such as code words and sign language. It's the dealer who is exposed. If the dealer is arrested, he can only inform on the go-between, who has already pledged to suffer the legal consequences in exchange for *his* silence. And those in the past who haven't co-operated can now be found in protective custody or in a graveyard.

James plies his trade in much the same way most street-level dealers I've met do. There's no standing on a street corner soliciting business, like you'd see in some fanciful TV show. Instead he made some friends (mainly through work) in Toronto and, after developing a modicum of two-way trust, let some of them know he was a user. With that barrier broken down, he introduced the idea of using together. The friends that agreed later became his customers. Then word got around and people started approaching him looking for meth. But, unless the person was properly introduced by an established customer, James denied any involvement with the drug. "You never know who's a cop," he said. "Or working for them."

Despite the fussy protocol, he never lacks for customers. He makes the rounds at various bars and clubs and will visit a buyer's home if he knows them well enough. Most of his customers, he says, are gay men ranging in age from nineteen to forty and almost all are involved with the club scene. When we talk about the ill effects of meth, he downplays the ones he doesn't deny completely. I attribute that to the fact that he's sitting beside a regular customer at the same table.

The Canadian model is roughly the same way meth gets distributed throughout much of the world except East Asia. The bikers recruit the cooks, the cooks make meth locally, the bikers sell it to middlemen and the middlemen find dealers. It's also the way it traditionally worked across much of the United States, and still does in pockets of the Midwest, especially in truck stops and small towns connected by highways.

But since 2002 (or a year later in more remote places), the number of meth labs busted has declined dramatically. "Yes, drastically down, in fact," said John Fernandes of the DEA. "Unfortunately there is an explosion of meth use." Indeed, the number of arrests for meth possession and the percentage of people who admit to meth use in surveys have not really declined anywhere and have risen in many places. The simple fact is that fewer and fewer people are making meth in the United States. The reasons aren't complicated, but they are numerous. Manufacturing meth is a dangerous business to begin with. Crackdowns have made accessing supplies and ingredients more difficult. Improved police detection and surveillance techniques have made manufacturing an even more fitful undertaking. Most important, however, has been competition from the Mexicans.

Although there have been a number of significant arrests in meth-related organized crime in Mexico—most notably the top of the Arrellano Brothers cartel—the volume of drugs coming north has increased. According to Gene Haislip, the DEA agent who led the original charge against meth, the product from the Mexican super-labs is usually about twice as pure as what can be achieved in a Beavis and Butt-head lab. Mexican labs employ large-scale round-the-clock production, and are rarely—if ever—hampered by police investigations, or drug legislation. They are better equipped, as well, to control and keep the incidence of fires and explosions to a minimum. Their supply chain is, therefore, virtually constant—something local labs can't come close to and an important consideration with a drug that is often used frequently.

Of course, transportation and border interdiction can cause problems, but the super labs counter them by using thousands of the illegal immigrants who regularly pass into the United

States as mules. There are simply so many of them that they can't all (or even a significant fraction of them) be caught. When the super labs were still located in California's Central Valley, border crossings could be easily identified by the massive piles of little white boxes of cold pills, hastily emptied so that their vital contents could be smuggled across more easily. Now that the labs have been relocated to Mexico, primarily around Guadalajara and Michoucan, the mountains of cardboard and tinfoil blister packs have mostly blown away. The smugglers, some of whom are "rewarded" into service and some of whom are simply threatened into it, now carry finished meth. Of course the penalties for the carriers are stiffer for carrying meth than they are for cold pills, but it really doesn't matter to the cartels who are virtually never informed on and have no shortage of people willing to take the risk. Considering that the U.S. Border Patrol found the bodies of 463 would-be immigrants in 2005 and tens of thousands are jailed every year, the process is already dangerous enough that just carrying a small amount of drugs really doesn't change many minds. According to the U.S. Department of Justice, U.S. attorneys prosecuted an increased number of non-citizens for other crimes, especially for drug trafficking, which increased from 1799 cases in 1985 to 7803 in 2000.

While illegal immigrants have traditionally looked for agricultural and service jobs in the U.S., more and more are trying to make a quick buck in the meth trade. Detective Mario Anaya of the Merced County Sheriff's office in California's Central Valley was investigating the murder of a migrant laborer, whose body was discovered at an abandoned lab on Deadman's Creek. The body had five gunshot wounds and was discovered among a pile of empty propane containers and sheets (most likely used as filters) stained with meth. The half-pound of finished meth and the $2000 in cash found at the scene indicated that the killers were unsophisticated and/or in a big hurry. On the walls of the lab were the words "stay out if you value your ass!" in both Spanish and English. "Farm labor is a dangerous occupation," said Anaya. "Unfortunately, they are trading that job for an even more dangerous one."

Once in the U.S., the mules meet up with a contact, invariably Mexican and well-known or related to cartel members back home. Although there are other groups involved, most of the contacts are members of the Mexican Mafia, also known as La Eme. Founded in a California prison not far from the Central Valley in 1950, the Mexican Mafia was originally intended to protect Mexican prisoners from the vicious black and white gangs who fought for dominance in the prison system. But like most groups of men who meet while incarcerated, it quickly turned into a criminal enterprise.

Once released, members of the Mexican Mafia used extortion against Mexican drug dealers operating in the U.S. (they called it "the tax") and operated protection rackets targeting Mexican-owned businesses, primarily restaurants. A huge increase in illegal immigration led to an exponential increase in members of the Mexican Mafia and the organization began to broaden its goals. Starting in the middle 1960s, members of the Mexican Mafia began to import drugs into the U.S. It started gradually with a little bit of weed going to fellow members and other Mexicans, but rapidly increased until the Mexican Mafia became the primary source of marijuana for much of California. Enjoying an almost total code of silence among its members and operatives, the gang was rarely slowed down by police. As enterprising members began selling to whites (even working in connection with the avowedly racist and decidedly violent Aryan Brotherhood), profits soared. Years of continuous financial success led to expansion as the group swept throughout the southwestern U.S., reaching as far and into Texas. And, along with the aid of the major Mexican cartels the Mexican Mafia in the 1980s became a major source of cocaine—and later meth—for American users. "They're making quite a lot of money off of meth," said Sgt. Fuillermo Gonzalez of the Tijuana police. "They are pretty much using the same routes that they've used in the past with cocaine and with marijuana." Most authorities now agree that at least 80 percent of the meth sold in the U.S. comes from Mexico. One DEA agent rather famously estimated that meth trafficking brought more currency into Mexico's economy than any other source except petroleum. Evidence to that effect is piling up along the border. Police in San Diego, a primary border crossing, announced a 106 percent increase in seizures of meth from 2004 to 2005. Customs agents patrolling the twenty-four bridges from Mexico to Texas confiscated 1067 pounds of meth in 2003.

While the DEA has been working with Mexican authorities to arrest the leaders of meth-producing organizations there, there's a big difference between prisons in Mexico and the U.S. As *The New York Times* reported:

> [Osiel] Cárdenas, the leader of the Gulf Cartel, managed to keep control of his gang from inside Mexico's main maximum-security prison, La Palma. The Nuevo Laredo police department served almost entirely at his pleasure, federal law authorities said, helping not only protect the Gulf Cartel, but also kidnapping and killing suspected rivals. And a group of special forces officers, known as Los Zetas, who had deserted from the military and served as Mr. Cárdenas' personal security detail when he was out of prison, were deployed to protect the Gulf Cartel's turf—especially Nuevo Laredo.

A significant advantage the Mexicans have, apparently, is their ferocity.

"For whatever reason," said a California cop I know, "whenever the Mexicans and the bikers came into confrontation, the bikers would run. I guess the bikers had more to lose, or other ways of making money." In any event, the Mexicans tend to be well armed. Police in Fresno, California, say that every time they bust a group of Mexican gangsters they find at least one semiautomatic weapon or worse. "These guys are packing big heat," said Robert Pennal, who leads the Fresno police's meth task force. "It's not so much to engage law enforcement as it is to protect their labs from being ripped off by rivals."

As more and more of the meth being sold in the United States flows from Mexico, the bikers have either been frozen out, moved to more remote and less-profitable areas of the trade, or been forced to work with the Mexicans. According to a report to Congress by George J. Cazenavette III, special agent in charge of the DEA's New Orleans office, "the increased power and sophistication of the Mexican traffickers led them to seek to successfully dominate all phases of the methamphetamine trade, from beginning to end."

More recently, outlaw motorcycle gangs—predominantly, but not entirely the Hells Angels—have been working in concert with the Mexican Mafia, selling their meth in smaller, more remote towns. It makes perfect sense for both sides. The Mexicans provide top quality meth and the Hells Angels supply a peerless distribution system and infrastructure. Not surprisingly, the alliance got its start in prison. According to the DEA's Drug Threat Assessment of 2003, "incarcerated Hells Angels members developed strong criminal ties to Mexican traffickers in prison. These associations facilitated the expansion of their methamphetamine production and distribution networks." Even in those parts of the U.S. where a Mexican national might raise suspicions or have a hard time making connections, Mexican drugs still arrive through more traditional and less conspicuous means on a Harley-Davidson.

And it's not just the bikers. Las Vegas perfectly fits the description of a meth-ravaged city. It has a largely white, lower- or middle-class population sprawled over a huge area. Much of its population is employed in low-paying service occupations, and many are working untraditional shifts and long hours. According to DEA agent Mike Flanagan, meth trafficking arrests are a daily occurrance.

"These meth organizations in Mexico are large-scale type organizations," he said. "They transport it here into the United States and then it goes to different cells."

The cells, he said, range from anonymous street-level dealers to some of the biggest and most powerful gangs in the U.S.

Although the Mexican Mafia traditionally disdains working with African-American criminal organizations, huge economic opportunities have trumped racism. The dominant meth suppliers in Las Vegas are Mexican, but the biggest dealers are black. The Rolling 60s are an established Los Angeles gang closely associated with the Crips organization and are the main retailers of meth in Las Vegas and surrounding Clark County, according to gang researcher Billy James Nolen. The gang migrated to Nevada quite recently, he said, but established a foothold very quickly.

But while Las Vegas—traditionally home to many types of organized crime and owner of an anything-goes reputation—may seem like a natural target for the Mexican Mafia, it's hardly alone. The Ozark Mountains of Southeastern Missouri may be the last place you'd expect to see Mexican organized crime, but they're there. When local police noticed a surprisingly sudden and rapid decline in meth lab busts (the area had established itself as having the highest concentration of small-time cooks in the nation), they exulted at first that they had turned the tide against the drug. As they learned from informants, however, they realized their mistake. *They* hadn't put the labs out of business. Their suspicions were confirmed when graffiti—signature tags from Mexican gangs—began appearing spray-painted around the area.

The Mexicans had arrived.

Susan Swain moved to the town of Frisbee, Missouri, because she wanted to raise her kids away from the crime and violence of bigger cities. It didn't take long for her illusions to be shattered as, a few days after she moved in, a dozen or more police cars descended on the mobile home across the street from her house.

"It was really surprising to have it happen this close to our kids," she said. "There were a lot of police cars that showed up, and people were handcuffed; it's scary for your kids."

The police discovered about a pound of meth at the scene. "In a matter of sixty days we've taken in a total of nine pounds of methamphetamine in three separate incidents," said Sgt. Kevin Glaser of the Southeast Missouri Drug Task Force. And the men arrested inside (who were not cooks but street-level dealers) were illegal immigrants. Glaser said that's becoming increasingly more common. "They were approached by people from Mexico who said 'here's an opportunity to make money. Take these drugs back up sell them [in the U.S.],'" he said. "That's how a lot of these people work."

There may be up to 8.4 million undocumented Mexicans in the U.S,, according to the Pew Hispanic Center, a nonpartisan research organization that tracks data specific to Hispanic people in the U.S. Unlike bikers, who sport—often ostentatiously—the badges and distinctive "uniforms" at their membership, undocumented workers who are pushed into service as drug mules remain anonymous. They keep to themselves, communicate only with those they know and trust, and communicate in code. They are in every way completely indistinguishable from the millions of laborers who cross the border desperate for honest work.

A Florida cop I spoke with agreed with Glaser about how normally law-abiding immigrants can be coerced into helping the meth industry and mused about the difficulty of stemming the flow. "Illegals are everywhere and you can't tell which ones are involved [with meth] and who isn't," he said. "And you can't stop them unless you have just cause—they're getting away with it mostly because we don't know who they are."

HOW TO SPOT A METH LAB

- Strong smell that might resemble urine, or unusual chemical smell like ether, ammonia, or acetone.
- Little or no traffic during the day, but lots of traffic at extremely late hours.
- Extra efforts made to cover windows or reinforce doors.
- Residents never putting their trash out or burning all trash.
- Lab materials surrounding property (lantern fuel cans, red chemically stained coffee filters, clear glass jugs and duct tape).
- Vehicles loaded with trunks, chemical containers, or basic chemistry paraphernalia — glassware, rubber tubing, etc.
- Inhabitants smoking outside due to the fumes.
- Dying grass or plants in a particular area.
- Windows open all day/night, including winter
- Renters carrying in propane grill tanks, gas cans, tubing, glass canning jars, coolers.
- Trash left behind that includes coffee filters, lithium batteries, acetone, cold tablet packages, plastic hoses, iodine, and lye packages

Sources: Clandestine Laboratory Investigators Association, Portsmouth (N.H.) Police Department

CAGING THE BEAST: LAW ENFORCEMENT

BRAD DURFY IS one of the most media-savvy cops I have ever spoken to. A detective sergeant with the Ontario Provincial Police (OPP) Drug Enforcement Section, he is friendly, polite and well-spoken. He's cheerfully forthcoming about the arrests he and his team have made, but will not be steered off topic, will never speculate on anything and, like a smart suspect, will never, ever give you anything you could possibly use against him.

Durfy oversees much of the anti-drug efforts in southwestern Ontario. It's a place tailor-made for meth. Aside from a couple of medium-sized cities (Windsor and London, which have their own police forces), southwestern Ontario is decidedly rural, overwhelmingly white, extraordinarily boring and, of far more importance—out of the jurisdiction of laws limiting the sale of pseudoephedrine. Nor is there much in the way of monitoring hazardous chemicals, like anhydrous ammonia.

"If you drew a line from Middlesex County to the Bruce Peninsula, that would give you the area where most of Ontario's meth is made," he told me. "There's a lot of it in Stratford and Sarnia's something of a meth town now." The people in the territory he describes generally make their money off cattle, corn, wheat and petroleum, so it's not a huge surprise that the meth-making there has much more in common with what's been done in Western North America than the East.

"About ninety-eight percent of the cooks here use the Birch method—some people call it the Nazi method—which requires anhydrous ammonia," he said. ""They steal it from farmers." They don't seem to be having a difficult time getting the stuff. "We have an awareness campaign targeted to farmers and we're getting some response, but the anhydrous cooks eventually find easy targets and then it travels by word of mouth," said Durfy. "It's like that old shampoo commercial 'I told two friends and she told two friends...'"

And getting necessary quantities of pseudoephedrine hasn't proven to be much of a barrier for meth manufacturers either. Although there are no binding regulations in Canada, many pharmacists—even those not associated with MethWatch—will monitor the sales of over-the-counter remedies that contain meth's active ingredient. Enterprising cooks, however, have engineered ways around the restrictions. "They'll often shoplift what they need or boost it from a delivery truck," Durfy said. "When they do buy it, they go to a city and fan out, buying one or two boxes at a time from different pharmacies."

While much of Durfy's work is still taking down independent marijuana farms (what the people in the area call "grow ops"), he readily points out that meth is the second-most prominent illegal drug in his jurisdiction and becoming much more popular. Realizing that people are increasingly wary of statistics, he put it in a way that was pretty easy to relate to. "I was on the job for five years before we found our first lab on November 8, 2002," he told me. "And since then, we've found twenty-one." While twenty-one lab busts in a little more than three years may not sound like much to someone who lives in Missouri, Minnesota, Colorado or Alberta, Durfy's point is clear—meth-making is new to Southwestern Ontario, but quickly establishing itself. After a February 2002 raid in a number of small towns in the area resulted in twenty-five arrests and the seizure of $700,000 worth of meth in one day, even the OPP was shocked. "The drug problem has come to the small communities of Ontario," announced OPP Deputy Inspector Jim Hutchinson, who also said he was "surprised, and a little taken aback" at how many drugs were being traded in places not normally associated with any kind of crime, let alone drug trafficking. "I am dismayed to say this is the quantity and type of drugs we are seeing in small communities." Durfy wasn't too surprised, except that it happened in Elgin and Oxford counties, when previously meth had only been found in around Perth County, some distance to the west.

I wondered aloud if Durfy and the OPP weren't just finding meth labs because they started looking for them. Durfy assures me that's not the case.

"We followed what was happening the Western Canada and the United States," he said, pointing out that they'd been looking for clandestine meth labs in the area since the late 1990s. "We saw it coming—what happens in the United States usually happens up here after a while." In response to the expectation of more and more labs popping up, the OPP put together a twenty-six-officer meth lab dismantling crew from officers throughout the province. Each member must pass a three-week course that includes lessons on handling hazardous chemicals, fires and booby traps.

Much of what I learn from Durfy and other Ontario cops doesn't surprise me, but one thing he said did. The meth police confiscated in the province, he said, had no firm connection to organized crime.

"The people who are making it are the ones selling it," he said. "It's a crime of opportunity—users start making the drug for their own supply and then start selling it to finance their own habit."

In his experience, groups of three or four users pool their resources, make meth, take what they want and sell the excess for money to make more meth, although he admits "it might be different out where you are" in Toronto. He may have changed his opinion in September 2006 when dozens of Ontario Hells Angels were arrested in Operation Tandem. Many of them were caught with meth in their posscession.

Biker gangs—especially the Hells Angels—are said to have a near monopoly on the meth distribution in British Columbia. They also have networks in Ontario and other provinces as well. While no large-scale arrests have implicated Ontario bikers in meth cooking or distribution, there have been busts of people associated with gang members exporting and importing ephedrine and pseudoephedrine over the Ontario–Michigan border, as well as gang associates arrested for the importation of MDMA in the same area.

There has been no evidence that Mexican organized crime has been directly involved.

In June 2006, however, just before the Mexican national election, the bodies of four federal drug officers were found (one without his head) with a sign reading *so you learn respect* in Acapulco, a resort city on the Pacific coast with a long history of connections to Canadian Hells Angels. A week earlier, three other drug officers and a man believed to be an informant were beheaded in Tijuana and their heads were dumped miles from their bodies.

What bothers cops I have spoken with is the interesting criticism that by busting local labs and dealers, law enforcement is simply clearing the market for organized crime to sweep in and take over. "What do they expect?" an exasperated Saskatchewan cop told me. "I don't have any jurisdiction in Mexico. If I find a guy who is risking his own life and those of the people around him to make an illegal and dangerous chemical, while at the same time destroying the environment, that I should just look the other way because some people believe he's keeping the Mexicans out?"

The truth is, if a cartel wants in, it will muscle its way in.

Whether it makes a difference or not, law enforcement at all levels has worked—and continues to work—very hard to bust meth labs. It isn't easy, but they have developed some reliable techniques. Two common methods police use to find meth labs, for instance, are informants—arrested meth users or dealers who exchange information for lighter sentences—and neighbors who either observe suspicious behavior or smell tell-tale odors (particularly the anhydrous ammonia required for the Nazi method or ether).

In November 2001, a woman in Lincoln, Nebraska, smelled a strange odor from a neighbor's house and gave the police an anonymous tip that she suspected he had a meth lab in his home. When the police arrived, they saw Randy Kleinholz and a friend relaxing on Kleinholz's porch. They smelled what they described as an "overpowering" scent of ether. The friend gave the cops permission to pat him down and was immediately arrested for possession of marijuana and drug paraphernalia. But Kleinholz did not consent. He argued with the police for about twenty minutes. He would not let them into the house and they would not let him in without an officer. They told him that the ether they smelled presented a danger to the public. He said that it wasn't ether, but, rather, some faulty plumbing.

The standoff ended when the police threatened to secure a search warrant. Frustrated, Kleinholz relented, and told the officers he would lead them into the house to show them the pipes that were the source of the odor. Inside the house, an officer pushed open a bedroom door and discovered a fully functional meth lab. Kleinholz was arrested.

When the case came to trial, the defense raised the issue of probable cause. The same issue was raised when the conviction was appealed.

In what may have been a ruling underscoring the state's conception of how serious the meth epidemic had become, the court ruled in favor of the police.

"The smell of ether might not alone support a finding of probable cause, but certainly such an odor coupled with other facts support a finding of probable cause," court ruled. "Due to the volatile nature of such labs, exigent circumstances justified an immediate but limited search." Nebraska cops made just one meth lab bust in 1999 The number had climbed to 365 by 2001.

Efforts to combat the meth plague through legislation are sharply on the rise. Some wonder if the efforts may not have reached "hysterical" proportions. In North Carolina in 2003 two district attorneys tried to have meth a declared a "weapon of mass destruction" and to be included under the state's antiterrorism law of 2001. One of the idea's proponents, District Attorney Jerry Wilson of Watauga County, wrote:

> Not only is the drug methamphetamine in itself a threat to both society and those using it, but the toxic compounds and deadly gases created as side products are also real threats. I feel that, as a prosecutor, I have to address this. Something has to be done to protect society.... I understand the title of the statute is antiterrorism, but the statute is much more broad than that. There's nothing in the statute that requires any organized terrorist effort. There's nothing in the statute that requires that these chemicals be used as a weapon.

One of Wilson's primary opponents, public defender Wallace Harrelson of Guildford County, replied:

> The law defines nuclear, biological or chemical weapons of mass destruction as, in part, 'any substance that is designed or has the capability to cause death or serious injury and is or contains toxic or poisonous chemicals or their immediate precursors.' It seems to me to be a real stretch of the imagination, that this would be covered under the antiterrorism law. It seems to me that the antiterrorism law was designed with a specific purpose in mind, to prosecute people who are threatening to hurt the safety of the general public.

Wilson was frank about his intentions. Anyone caught violating the antiterrorism law's weapons of mass destruction section, he said, would be liable to twelve years to life in prison for each count, while the existing sentencing guidelines for meth manufacture in North Carolina recommended far less stiff penalties—usually about six months for an uncomplicated first offense.

Wilson's first use of the antiterrorism legislation against meth makers came with the arrest of twenty-four-year-old Martin Dwayne Miller who lived just outside the town of Todd. Miller was held for months in lieu of a $505,000 bond until his trial began. Unfortunately for Wilson, his test case scenario hit a bump right out of the gate.

Watauga County Superior Court Judge James Baker stated that the charges against Miller were vague and, therefore, violated his rights outlined by the Fourteenth Amendment to the U.S. Constitution, which provide protection from government's overzealous application of law and punishment. He also made it clear in his decision that if the enactors of the law had intended to include clandestine drug labs under the legislation, they would have specifically written them into the text.

Wilson and others after him ultimately failed to have meth legally declared—for prosecution purposes—a weapon of mass destruction, but a more narrowly defined version of his bill emerged.

When it was introduced and later passed through the U.S. Senate by a 98-1 vote and through the House 357-66, the Uniting and Strengthening America by Providing Appropriate Tools Required to Intercept and Obstruct Terrorism Act of 2001 (better known as the USA Patriot Act or Public Law 107-56) was considered controversial. Signed into law less than seven weeks after the 9/11 terrorist attacks on the World Trade Centers and the Pentagon, the USA Patriot Act immediately drew criticism for its apparent violations of any number of civil liberties. In question particularly were Section 215, which allowed Federal Bureau of Investigation (FBI) agents to secure search warrants *in camera* (in secret) from the United States Foreign Intelligence Surveillance Court for library or bookstore records and receipts for anyone suspected to be connected with terrorism or spying, and Section 213, which allowed the FBI to employ what the officers themselves called "sneak-and-peek" powers—the ability to acquire search warrants or the equivalent thereof *after* the actual search.

Two senators from meth-plagued states, Democrat Dianne Feinstein of California and Republican Jim Talent of Missouri, had been developing a federal anti-meth bill, which would impose nationwide limits on the sale of pseudoephedrine. They cited statistics that similar restrictions had led to a large and rapid decline in the number of meth labs shut down in states like Arkansas, Oregon and Missouri. Their bill was gathering broad support, and in the spring of 2005 it was announced that the meth restrictions would be made a provision of the revised USA Patriot Act, to be put into law the following September.

Under the new law, anyone in the U.S. must produce picture identification to purchase products containing pseudoephedrine, and each person would be limited to three hundred 30 mg doses of pseudoephedrine with a maximum purchase of 120 in a single day. It also meant that the chemical had to be kept behind the counter and locked in pharmacies, could not be sold in flea market-type venues or by mail order and the old "blister pack" packaging was banned. It also committed $495 million in federal funds over five years to train meth-lab investigators. There was nothing in the bill for increased penalties, relaxed search warrants or methods or extra powers for investigators.

Both sides of the House congratulated themselves on the new law.

"By signing this bill, President Bush and Congress struck a blow against a different kind of terrorist, those who produce and sell meth," said Chris Cannon, a Republican from Utah. "This bill will help reduce supply and stiffen existing penalties for those who deal in this dangerous drug."

Not surprisingly, the Democrats were somewhat less effusive in their praise.

"I'm pleased that we came up with this bi-cameral, bi-partisan resolution that recognizes that we need to deal with the meth problem on two fronts—domestically and internationally," said Leonard Boswell, a Democrat from Iowa.

Those in the law enforcement community hailed the very idea of a nationwide pseudoephedrine restriction as a triumph. "If we leave it up to local jurisdiction, we're simply going to move the problem from one jurisdiction to another without addressing the root cause," said Jerry Dyer, chief of the Fresno, California, police. He also detailed the traditional scenario of what happened when a state or community within the U.S. had passed similar statutes: as pseudoephedrine becomes more scarce in the area, black market prices for it rise. And when the prices get high enough, the cooks simply find another supply in a neighboring jurisdiction. But with a nationwide law in place, those neighboring jurisdictions are off limits. The only source becomes importation from foreign countries. While pseudoephedrine can, and has, come from Mexico and Canada, it's not an easy process and defeats one of the most alluring aspects of the meth trade—cooks never had to depend on the whims of foreign suppliers as had those who sold coke, crack, MDMA or any of a number of other drugs.

The amount of pseudoephedrine imported to the U.S. from Mexico has effectively dropped to nothing. While recent crackdowns on the importation of the chemical and its retail sale in Mexico may have had something to do with that, so did increased border surveillance and interdiction operations by U.S. agents. In the middle-1990s, two DEA-led campaigns— Operations Mountain Express I and II—led to the arrest of 189 suspected smugglers and the seizure of 12.5 tons of pseudoephedrine, 83 pounds of actual finished methamphetamine and $11.1 million in U.S. currency. Although they certainly didn't shut down the Mexican cartels, they did change their strategy. Instead of importing pseudoephedrine to labs in California, the gangsters moved their manufacturing to Mexico and began importing finished product only.

Canada has no nationwide laws limiting the retail sale of pseudoephedrine, but some meth-affected provinces like Alberta and Nova Scotia have provincial restrictions and others are contemplating legislation. What Canada does have is a law— called the Precursor Control Regulations—which came into effect in a series of stages from January 9, 2003 to January 1, 2004. But while they do place strong restrictions on the import, export, manufacture and repackaging of such chemicals, they make no reference to retail sale. Basically, anyone in most of

Canada can buy as much pseudoephedrine as they want. And the feds have long been of aware of this.

"In Canada the pseudoephedrine is not regulated, and so it is lawful to load up a semi-trailer truckload in Canada of pseudoephedrine," said DEA Asa Hutchinson. "It is illegal to bring it in the United States when it is going in to illegal purposes."

In January 2002, the DEA announced the conclusion of Operation Mountain Express III, a campaign that targeted illegal pseudoephedrine importation from Canada. The magnitude of the bust was alarming. In 2000, the entire nation of Canada imported fifty-five tons of pseudoephedrine from all sources and for all reasons and in a single operation, the DEA intercepted sixteen tons coming to the U.S. from Canada in one operation. If all of the pseudoephedrine had been properly cooked, it could have been used to make 37,000 pounds of meth. That's more than six times the total seized by the feds in the United States in all of 2001!

U.S. Customs Service Commissioner Robert Bonner described the first seizure to the press:

The first of the eight seizures occurred on April 11th of 2001, and it was a particularly brazen attempt to smuggle a huge amount of pseudoephedrine into the United States. A truck driver arrived at the Port of Detroit with a shipping manifest claiming that the truck was empty. And, by the way, that's not unusual to have empties coming back across the border. But the manifest said this truck was empty. And, despite that, the very alert Customs inspector decided to order that truck over to what's called secondary inspection. And inside the truck he found 43 million tablets of pseudoephedrine packed in about... roughly about twelve tons of pseudoephedrine. The stash was more than large enough to convince the Customs inspector that these drugs were going to be used for something other than to treat colds. In fact, I think there was enough decongestant in that— that one truck itself to unplug about every nose in Michigan for several years.

Typically, the smugglers would rent (or, more often, steal) a tractor-trailer and had the audacity to paint Federal Express or even U.S. Postal Service logos on them to thwart detection. The trucks were then intended to meet up with organized crime groups once they were past the border. About half were aligned with the Jafar Organization in Detroit and the rest went to the Yassaoui Brothers in Chicago. The DEA had not ignored the fact that both gangs had leadership connections with roots in the Middle East.

"The majority of the traffickers are of Middle Eastern descent, and we have determined that they send drug proceeds in part back to the Middle East," said Hutchinson. "And we are continuing to follow the money trail." No direct connection to any terrorist activity was ever announced, though.

A similar sting—Operation Northern Star—in which sixty-five people were arrested in places as disparate as Los Angeles, Ottawa and Gulfport, Mississippi, went down the following year. Six of the arrested suspects turned out to be top executives from three Canadian pharmaceuticals firms—G.C. Medical Products, Formulex and Frega—who personally sold huge amounts of pseudoephedrine to Americans for illegal use. According to the DEA:

One company, Frega, Inc. is charged criminally in Detroit for its role in supplying bulk quantities of pseudoephedrine to brokers in Cincinnati and Chicago. Approximately 14,000 pounds (108 million tablets) of

pseudoephedrine originating from Frega, Inc. was
seized during this investigation. This pseudoephedrine,
believed to be destined for meth labs in the western
United States, would yield approximately 9,000 pounds
of methamphetamine with a street value of between
$36 million and $144 million.

Again, the bulk of the contacts on the U.S. side were involved
in recognized organized crime groups, and many of them were
again, the DEA asserted, of Middle Eastern descent. Interestingly,
police from the island nation of Cyprus made two arrests.

Hundreds of thousands of people cross between Canada
and the U.S. every day, many of them at Detroit and other
Ontario crossings with U.S. cities on or close to the other side
like Sault Ste. Marie, Sarnia, Fort Erie, Niagara Falls, Kingston
and Cornwall. In the almost one hundred times I've crossed the
border by car, I have been stopped once—when my license plate
number matched that of a car reported to have been stolen. My
car was a white Nissan and the stolen car in question was a black
Mercedes-Benz, so I was waved across after ten minutes.

In truth, only a very tiny fraction of a percent of border
crossers is ever stopped. Even fewer are searched. Those that are
usually give the Customs officials a reason to do so, although
often involuntarily through visual or behavioral cues. Smart
smugglers are aware of this, and work to look as inconspicuous
as possible. A wig to cover a shaved head, long sleeves to cover
up a tattoo, and your garden variety tweaker cook transforms
into a regular guy.

I asked him Durfy about whether meth or pseudoephedrine
was being traded over the border.

"I can't easily comment on that sort of thing. I wouldn't want
to endanger any current or future investigations."

GOING
UNDERGROUND

THE FIRST THING I noticed about Justin when I first met him face-to-face was his breath. He had that acrid breath that irritates the linings of your nostrils and makes you want to inhale through your mouth. It's his teeth—or what's left of them. Justin has an advanced case of what some dentists and many in the media are calling "meth mouth"—rapid disintegration of the user's teeth caused by meth use.

He's not alone.

Dr. Brett Kessler is a dentist with a thriving practice in Stapleton, the giant planned community that occupies the space where Denver's first international airport stood until it was decommissioned in 1995. On his off-hours, Kessler volunteers at Sobriety House, Denver's oldest substance-abuse treatment center, providing free dental work to its clients. Much of his work—more than fifty cases—has been devoted to reversing or at least reducing the effects of meth mouth, which he still finds disturbing after twelve years in practice.

"It's just devastating," he said. "It's a scary smile." Excessive tooth decay is not just about having an attractive smile. Tooth breakage and loss can be an exceptionally painful experience.

"One patient would get high and pull his own tooth," said Kessler. "He'd get high again to kill the pain."

It can have other nasty effects. Catherine Okoro, an epidemiologist working for the Centers for Disease Control (CDC) published a report in the *American Journal of Preventive Medicine* that links tooth loss to heart attacks. After adjusting for such variables as sex, race and ethnicity, education, marital status, diabetes, smoking status, alcohol consumption, high blood pressure, high blood cholesterol and body mass index, Okoro reported that an increase in the number of lost teeth has a direct correlation to the risk of heart attack.

Meth addicts suffer from accelerated tooth decay primarily due to a reduction of the amount of saliva in the mouths. Xerostomia is the medical term for what most people call "dry mouth." Although there can be medical causes—most often diabetes or blocked salivary ducts—we most often do it to ourselves. Dry mouth is usually the side effect of the use or over-use of alcohol, certain medications like decongestants, marijuana or other drugs. Few people have ever woken up after a drinking binge or a few joints and not suffered from a mouth that felt like it was full of absorbent cotton. The problem can be made much worse by the fact that meth users often sleep with their mouths open after binges—because the body sleeps more deeply and needs more oxygen.

The effects are more than just an unpleasant feeling and bad breath. Reduced saliva production removes teeth's protection from contaminants, especially at the gumline. Teeth begin to rot near their root and quickly break or fall out. Otherwise healthy teeth next to the damaged or lost ones become affected either by same contaminants or through overuse.

Many meth users exacerbate the problem by smoking tobacco and/or marijuana—both of which are very effective saliva inhibitors. They make matters worse by fighting dry mouth with huge amounts of sugary soft drinks, which a tweaking body craves.

Justin prefers orange soda.

Meth, as a powerful vasocontrictor, can also reduce the amount of blood flow to the gums and surrounding bone. This can lead to periodontitis, also known as pyorrhea, which is a condition in which plaque below the gumline contributes to loss of bone tissue in the area surrounding the teeth. As the bone around them is gradually weakened and reduced, teeth become loose and eventually fall out.

While high, the users of stimulants also often grind or clench their teeth. Although these symptoms are more closely associated with MDMA (ecstasy), they are also common among meth users. The clenching, which doctors call trisma, is a result of involuntary spasms of the jaw muscles and the user is often unaware that it's happening. The grinding, or bruxia, is similar, but is the result of a different set of muscles, those that move the mandible from side to side. The strain from either can severely damage teeth, especially those already in states of decay.

While all of these factors contribute to tooth damage and loss, most citations of meth mouth in the media indicate that lifestyle habits—poor diet, a relaxed attitude towards basic hygiene and a lack of visits to dental professionals—play an important if not primary role in tooth decay among meth users.

It's pure conjecture how many meth addicts are concerned about their appearance and odour, but I'd bet some—especially users whose habits have not advanced that far, might be. Many meth users I have spoken with have regular jobs and sex lives that would be adversely affected by poor hygiene. Four of the Canadian users I mentioned earlier—Brian, Kyle, James and

Taylor—dress cleanly if not always tastefully, appear clean and well groomed. They brush, floss and even see dentists (although perhaps not as often as they should). Taylor has what appear to be above-average teeth, but the guys showed signs of advancing dental decay. It was only a matter of time.

An odd and some might say an ultimately trivial battle has erupted—a battle that has severely divided people on the meth issue and led to accusations of grandstanding, scare-mongering and blowing the problem out of proportion. Media—particularly daily newspapers—in many areas hit hard by meth, have been regularly promoting the notion that meth mouth is caused by, or helped along by, toxins in the meth itself. The theory is that some of the elements used in making meth—like anhydrous ammonia, lye and lithium—make it an acidic compound that destroys teeth.

Opponents counter that none of those elements are acids, but neglect to mention that ammonia and lye can be just as corrosive as any acid. It's hard to imagine why, ultimately, it matters. In any case, conventional wisdom suggests it's unlikely any meth ingredient leads to tooth decay from direct contact.

"There is speculation about the possibility that the drug itself directly produces some of the tooth destruction since it is somewhat caustic by itself," said Dr. Martin S. Spiller, a dentist who practices in Townsend, Maryland. "However, the drug is in direct contact with the teeth for only a very short time and is quite water-soluble." If there are any corrosive elements in the meth, they are washed away before they can do any damage. Many also cite Dr. John R. Richard's article in the August 2000 *Journal of Periodontology*, in which he details a study of forty-nine meth users and found that those with purer meth suffered just as much tooth damage as those with the suspect adulterants.

What may be more relevant is the question of whether the media is telling the whole truth about why it's happening. After working in newspapers, magazines and other media for almost two decades, I've seen how these things happen. Reporters generally don't lie to push agendas (particularly ones that agree with police and government). Instead they are overworked, pressed by deadlines or just plain lazy enough to simply repeat what they are told, especially if the source is considered reliable. On the front page of the *The New York Times*, on June 11, 2005, an article about meth mouth contained this passage:

> Other dentists said they suspected that the caustic ingredients of the drug—whether smoked, injected, snorted or eaten—contributed to the damage, which tends to start near the gums and wander to the edges of teeth. Among ingredients that can be used to make meth are red phosphorus found in the strips on boxes of matches and lithium from car batteries.

It's a remarkably short jump from *The Times* saying some dentists suspect something to a local paper reporting it as fact (although I feel obligated to mention that lithium doesn't come from car batteries). It's a concept known in the business as echo-chamber journalism. If a reporter hears something often enough, especially from other reporters, he or she begins to believe it's a fact and reports it as such.

But the argument isn't about whether the anhydrous ammonia used to make meth causes tooth decay or not. It's about whether the media is giving an accurate picture of what's happening with the drug, who it's affecting and if it's getting worse or not. Much of the controversy began after *Newsweek* published a cover package on meth anchored by a lead story by Paul R. Jefferson called "America's Most Dangerous Drug." It was an all-encompassing article that used stories from users, police and government sources to indicate how awful the drug could be.

The backlash was immediate. Led by columnist Jack Shafer in *Slate* (which is actually owned by the same company as *Newsweek*, weakening the oft-repeated accusation that reporters write stories to please their corporate overlords), many found fault with the whole package. In an essay called "Meth Madness at *Newsweek*: This Is Your Magazine on Drugs," Shafer criticized Jefferson for calling meth "the most dangerous drug," but not supplying a "body count." Instead, he points out that, in 2000, Los Angeles led U.S. cities with a mere 155 verified meth-related fatalities but fails to mention that it was a big jump from the 111 in the previous year and that statistics have risen nationwide in the five years since those figures were compiled. And I believe that it's actually a touch misleading to equate "dangerous" with fatal. Most meth users and addicts don't die from the drug, but they and their families, associates, employers and communities certainly do suffer.

Shafer also describes the billions of amphetamine pills that were legally produced and distributed in the U.S. for decades before they were controlled. "Those pills," he writes, "were potentially just as addictive and potentially just as deadly as the meth found on the street today." He may believe that, but I don't know anyone—doctor, user, cop, cook, politician or dealer—who agrees with him.

According to 1992 study by Dr. Jeff Winger at Mississippi State University, methamphetamine has a much more profound affect on the human central nervous system because it penetrates further and because of its longer half-life. Journalists have frequently based their stories on the belief that amphetamines and methamphetamines are interchangeable, neglecting—or conveniently forgetting—that they aren't. Not by a long shot. Amphetamines were considered dangerous by most doctors as early as 1949. Even when amphetamine was freely available over the counter, methamphetamine was a strictly controlled prescription drug.

The controversy has divided much of the media into two camps. Those who believe meth is bad, dangerous and rapidly spreading and those who believe meth is bad, dangerous and that the other guys are blowing it out of proportion. Dan Gardner is a respected and award-winning columnist for the *Ottawa Citizen*. In his piece "The Meth Epidemic That Isn't," he calls reporters who use opinions and statistics supplied by police and government "wide-eyed as toddlers and their reporting is little more than stenography." Instead, he bases his opinions on drug-use surveys, which he admits "aren't perfect," but are "fairly reliable." I'm not sure how he knows that, but in an effort to prove that meth isn't spreading and isn't becoming more popular, he cites an unnamed 2004 survey in which fewer Toronto students reported using meth than did in 1993. Interesting, but by no means definitive.

Almost all surveys that report a decline in meth use involve high school students—a group that has never been a big part of the meth community and are notoriously unreliable when it comes to drug-use surveys. It's been a long time, but I don't recall me or my friends ever telling the truth on them. And there are other surveys that say exactly the opposite. Besides, Toronto, outside of its gay community, has never had meth problem. It just doesn't fit the profile. A similar survey in Saskatoon or Edmonton or Stratford, Ontario, would no doubt have a very different result. If it asked the right people the right questions. And they answered honestly.

HOLLYWOOD-BASED writer Creighton Vero remembers being surrounded by meth users when he was enrolled at the University of Oregon in Eugene, and was surprised how little people in Los Angeles and New York knew about the drug. He thought it would be a good idea to make a documentary about the tweaker lifestyle, so he arranged some funding from Muse Films, an independent production house, and began to interview addicts. While most of them had little interesting to say, Vero found a guy named Will De Los Santos fascinating. Thin, hyperactive and unfailingly boastful, De Los Santos told him (in intricate detail) about his experiences driving a meth cook around Eugene for three days. Vero liked the story so much, he decided to ditch his documentary idea and make a narrative film based as closely as he could on De Los Santos' story.

Muse liked the picaresque idea and soon notable music video director Jonas Åkerlund and a troupe of talented actors attached themselves to the project. De Los Santos was given a co-writing credit, but was banned from the set, a technician who worked on the film told me, after his constant drug use became a distraction. With a $2.8 million budget, *Spun* was shot in and around Los Angeles in just twenty-two days.

The end result is a very entertaining film, pushed along by excellent performances by actors like John Leguizamo, Brittany Murphy, Jason Schwartzman and Mena Suvari. It's not for everyone, though. In an attempt to duplicate the frenetic, disjointed perspective of a meth user, Åkerlund used more than five thousand edits in the 101-minute film (a Hollywood record by a huge margin) and includes scenes that are as short as 0.083 seconds. Åkerlund did a great deal of research on the subject, talking to all kinds of users, dealers, cops and cooks. Although he declared that he met "very few people [in Oregon] who hadn't had a bad experience with meth," he always kept going back to De Los Santos' story. It didn't exactly fit the traditional cinematic story arc, but it was fascinating and informative. "If anything, in the editing process I was worried that we were too weird. The film starts out very strong. There's no climax," Åkerlund said. "If you went to film school and studied standard screenwriting, you'd say this is the wrong way to make a movie."

What happens to the characters in *Spun* is very much like what happens to actual meth users. When interviewed about the film long after its release, De Los Santos claimed that there were very few differences between what's represented in *Spun* and his actual experiences. He said that the inclusion of two comical, meth-addicted cops "were an embellishment on Åkerlund's part," but that every other "character in that movie is from my experiences." Aside from the cops, the changes from De Los Santos' memory to film were slight. The nude girl handcuffed to a motel bed for three days while Schwartzman's character drove the cook around was actually a nude girl tied to a motel bed for three hours with "strips of sheet and duct tape" while De Los Santos drove the cook around. That, and the names are changed.

But you won't see *Spun* mentioned in too many newspaper editorials. Despite its popular young stars, slick production values and edgy soundtrack, *Spun* is indisputably a cautionary and even frightening look at what meth does to people. In no way does it glamorize meth use or its manufacture, but it constantly warns about its dangers. "You want it to look cool, you want the audience to like the characters, but at the same time you hope it shows the ravages that drugs cause," said Åkerlund. "The film still works as an anti-drug statement."

THE MAIN POINT critics of media coverage of meth want to get across is that it's irresponsible and potentially dangerous for publications like *Newsweek* to whip up public antipathy for meth and its users. Very few people consider meth a good thing, but the writers of these opponent pieces believe that the hype surrounding a drug (or other perceived enemies of society) can lead to oppressive laws and their byproducts. Shafer wrote in his criticism of *Newsweek*:

This critique is no brief in favor of drug use. Nor do I minimize the collateral damage inflicted on others by methamphetamine users. But journalism like this ignores how, to paraphrase Grinspoon and Hedblom, drug-war measures often do more harm to individuals and society than the original "evil" substance the warriors attempted to stamp out.

But recent criticism leveled at the critics counters that they are not really aware of what they're talking about. While they quote statistics and survey numbers that support their opinions, their opponents point out that they rarely seem to talk with anyone who ever uses, cooks or sells the drug or (perhaps even more important) any doctor, social worker or anyone else who's had to help them. And when media reports about how meth use is not rising, spreading or prevalent come from places like New York or Toronto, it can make readers in other parts of the continent wonder if they know what's going on outside their largely meth-free cities. Whether it's an accurate opinion or not, many readers outside major Eastern media centers have told me that they consider those sorts of editorials more than a little naïve. As one cop said to me in parody: "Nobody in my family uses it, nobody at my country club uses it, so that obviously must mean that nobody's using it."

While it's clear that their desire is to prevent meth hype from leading politicians to grant extra powers to police and government, their critics say that by denying the meth epidemic, they are doing a great disservice to all the addicts who need help and all the care providers who need funding.

To his credit, Shafer quoted an e-mail sent to him by Richard A. Rawson, the well-known meth researcher from UCLA, in his *Slate* column:

Meth has been a major public health problem here
[southern California] almost twenty years. Data from
San Diego, one of the places with the longest standing
meth problems reported data about three months ago in
California. The problem there, according to all indicators is worse today than ever. Meth is not going away.
Once it gets into a community, it stays....

I wish people from New York and Washington who
think that meth is a pseudo problem would spend some
time in Indiana, Oregon, Oklahoma, Tennessee, etc. I
think if you talked with the workers in foster care programs, dentists, mental health workers, ob-gyns,
etc.—not politicians and police chiefs, trying to use the
hype for more funding—the real workers, you would
begin to wonder about the accuracy of the epidemiolog-
ical reports from East Coast experts.

While Jefferson, Shafer and Rawson are engaged in a spir-
ited debate, they are all lucid and respectable people who have
different views on how to achieve the same goal—limiting the
destruction caused by meth while retaining civil liberties. Not
everybody has the same desires.

In many of the same books and Web sites that offer meth
recipes, you'll find lots of specious reasoning and utterly outra-
geous nonsense. Among my favorites is the oft-repeated
statement that it's impossible to smell a meth user, contrary to
what cops claim. Instead, they reason, that what people smell is
fatigue, which forces the body to excrete chemicals. The fatigue,
they admit, comes from the fact that meth makes the user stay
up for three or four days of manic activity. They also generally
point out that the pungency of a tweaker comes from the ammonia in the drug. At the same time, the claim is made that none
of the toxic constituent agents in meth, such as ammonia, are

BUYER BEWARE

Paul and Cynthia Halliday scraped together every cent they had to buy a house. To the recently married couple, the cute little brick bungalow in Orem, Utah, was the first step towards the fulfillment of their shared desires. He was longing to get out of the student dorm at Brigham Young University and she really wanted to start a family.

Soon after they moved in, a neighbor came over and told the Hallidays about the previous resident, a tenant who hosted a huge number of parties, had visitors at all hours and disappeared without warning. Alarmed, Cynthia had the building tested for meth contamination. She was stunned by the results. The Hallidays' dream house contained 70 times the maximum allowable amount of toxic chemicals, all them associated with meth manufacture.

Forced by state authorities to move out, the Hallidays claim that they have lost "furniture, clothes, electronics, a piano, other musical instruments, photographs, heirlooms, tools, sports equipment" — basically everything they own — because of the contamination. They also say the five month they spent in the house has led them to experience "frequent headaches, diarrhea, shortness of breath, skin rashes and chronic coughing and has put them at risk of cancer, liver damage and damage to the reproduction system."

Cynthia, who has since discovered that she's pregnant, has filed suit against Osmond Real Estate for, among other things, concealing the knowledge that the house was uninhabitable. Osmond Real Estate was founded by George Osmond, father of Donny and Marie, in 1979 and is now overseen by their younger brother Jimmy.

Source: Salt Lake Tribune

ingested by the meth user, having been transformed or disposed of in the cooking process. So, to sum it up: meth users don't smell, except they do and the smell is ammonia leaking from their bodies, except they don't actually ingest any ammonia. It's the kind of self-deluded rationalization designed to make a meth user feel better about him- or herself.

And the debate rages on. But setting aside for a moment those purposes people will use any writing for, some ideas that can be accepted as fact remain. Meth is extremely dangerous, with prolonged use resulting in brain damage and other ailments. Meth is highly addictive, although that addiction is perhaps not so quick to set in as the DEA would have us believe. Meth users put strains, sometimes in colossal proportions, on friends, families, communities, law enforcement, the environment, the medical system and other care givers.

But what's in question is how many people are using it, whether there more or less of them and whether meth is spreading into areas and communities where it couldn't be found before. It's impossible to answer those questions without somebody producing a statistic or a survey or an expert to contradict your opinion.

It's just the nature of illegal activity to be covert and clandestine and not respond honestly to surveys. What statistics we can collect are arrest records, hospital admission records and rehab facility files. They do not reflect the users—perhaps the majority—who are never arrested, hurt or try to give up. There's simply no way to determine any accurate numbers representing drug use without a little faith or fudging.

I can't tell you how many people are using meth, but when I started looking for them, there were way more than I thought there would be. And, perhaps more importantly, I found plenty of meth users in places where I had not encountered any in previous years. It may not be spreading across the continent like the "prairie fire" or "brush fire" some say it is, but meth exists in large amounts where it didn't ten years ago and is, from my experience, being used by people who wouldn't have if they encountered it a generation ago.

Whether meth use is an epidemic depends on your definition of the word. If you think that meth use would qualify as an epidemic because its use is widespread and growing, because it has had a profound effect on culture, law enforcement, the medical community, our shared economy and public policy and because it's dangerous and unnecessary, then I would hasten to agree with you. And, from my research, I believe all of those things are true.

"DO YOU KNOW WHERE YOUR CHILDREN ARE?"

I'M IN A DREARY Tim Horton's near one of Toronto's busiest intersections on a Saturday night and I'm surprised at how dead it is. It's a big place and there's hardly anyone here, despite a lot of pedestrian traffic on the street outside. But if you watch closely enough, you can always see some drama. At a table right near the front, there's a nice-looking young man, leaning back in his seat. He smiles at everyone who comes in. He says "hi" to me with a sardonic grin and an affected lisp. He's selling something, maybe drugs. I grab a coffee, sit down and wait for Brian to show up. In the meantime, I observe as the four middle-aged men in the shop, all sitting alone and sneaking glances at the younger man, slowly gather up the nerve to approach him.

Brian finally arrives, and he's angry. A friend of his was arrested for cocaine possession and is now very likely to go to prison. "It sucks, it totally sucks, he's a great guy, too," he told me. "They should just legalize it, then there wouldn't be any more crime." I ask him if he feels the same way about meth and he told me something I think is pretty significant.

"Yeah, people should be allowed to make their own mistakes."

IN FEBRUARY 2006, Arizona criminal defense attorney Marc Victor became the first recognized credible voice to support the legalization of meth. He's an unlikely advocate for legislation. A self-described "health nut," he eats only organic foods and visits the gym six times a week. He has three children and says that the last thing he wants any of them to be is a drug addict. Reasons for maintaining the status quo for him are blissfully pragmatic. "As a practicing criminal defense attorney, I make a good income from defending people who are charged with drug crimes," he said. "If the drug war ended, I would lose a substantial portion of my income."

It's not that he is—as some in the media are—downplaying the dangers of meth.

"The question is not whether meth is dangerous and unhealthy," he writes. "Over the years, I have represented countless meth users. I have seen the consequences of meth use up close. I am convinced meth use will likely ruin the user's life. It is an extraordinarily dangerous addictive drug. Few drugs are more addictive or dangerous than meth. Many of those who oppose legalization of meth identify the horrors of meth use. I entirely agree with their assessment of meth's dangers."

His seemingly paradoxical opinion on meth (it's terrible stuff, but it should be available) stems from his opinion—shared by many people, including Brian—that legalizing meth would be for the common good. His argument is based on two points: a) the government has no right to tell people what they should and should not do to their own bodies and b) if the government regulated the manufacture, sale and purity of meth it would eliminate the organized crime associated with it, as well

as protect users by ensuring what they got was free of dangerous impurities.

He certainly has a point with the freedom argument.
Suppose we replace the word "meth" with "meat." According to
an opinionated segment of the population, the consumption of
meat is addictive. They also say it's bad for your health and terrible for the environment. Try to imagine, however, anyone
anywhere taking seriously a ban on the consumption of meat.

Milton Friedman, the respected economist and an outspoken
critic of the war on drugs, has made a more nuanced argument.
"I believe that there is a case for keeping certain things out of the
market," he writes. "I believe it's not desirable to have a market
in atomic bombs. But the number and the list of things for which
you can really justify prohibition is very limited. And the only jus-
tification is always in terms of the existence of innocent victims,
not in terms of paternalistic concern."

The question, if you agree with Friedman, would then
appear to be whether meth affects those other than its voluntary
users—is it meat or an atomic bomb? The children of meth
addicts suffer; the same could be said, however, for the children
of alcoholics. Drunk driving injuries and fatalities—especially
when measured against innocent victims—far outnumber those
caused by meth abuse.

On the other hand, alcohol and nicotine have been bedrock
parts of our shared Western culture for about 9000 and 500
years, respectively. So much are they entwined in the fabric of
our culture that previous and periodic efforts by government to
suppress them have been themselves failures. True, the popularity of alcohol remains basically constant, while smoking tobacco
is on the wane, at least in the West.

The opposite is occurring with marijuana. Downgraded to a
misdemeanor in many parts of North America, weed is gaining
in its number of users and advocates. Although there have been

no conclusive studies, marijuana is normally considered by the scientific community to be less likely to cause emphysema or cancer, even among heavy smokers, than tobacco. Popularly, it is considered almost antithetical to violence and is rarely linked to any crime other than its own possession, importation or sale.

As more and more people use marijuana, governments are forced to submit to public will and relax laws or at least penalties associated with its use. Widespread decriminalization of weed has taken root in places like the Netherlands, Colorado, Ontario and Massachusetts. At the same time, tobacco use is under widespread assault. Increasingly, restrictive legislation—as well as costly liability litigation—has the industry reeling on its heels, at least in North America. Weirdly, as tobacco use inches toward illegality, marijuana use is bounding towards official acceptance.

Smokers are being demonized—but not pot smokers.

Meanwhile, the conventional stereotype of an addle-headed pot smoker is being revised and has become increasingly positive. While most people's image of an overindulging pothead is that of a lazy but amiable burnout with a penchant for Doritos—not that far off from the lovable town drunk of a generation or so ago—every tobacco smoker has the image of a lung cancer patient, wheezing and gasping for their final breath burned into their consciousness. But marijuana's image appears to be rapidly improving. Entertainers Robert Altman, Jennifer Aniston, Jack Black, Harrison Ford, Matthew McConaughey, Bill Murray and Brad Pitt have all admitted to having smoked pot. Adding even more credence to the idea that marijuana is an acceptable alternative to alcohol or nicotine use is the evidence that politicians such as Bill Clinton, Al Gore, Pierre Trudeau, Newt Gingrich, Michael Bloomberg and others have also tried it. (Even revered statesmen like George Washington, Winston Churchill and Thomas Jefferson are believed by some to have gotten high. It doesn't matter if they did or not; what's important is that many people *believe* that they did.)

No politician, no star, no celebrity, however, is wiling to cheerfully confess to recreational meth use.

NO STAR WAS BETTER known and better loved in her time than Judy Garland. The tiny singer with the big voice was born Francis Gumm, but was better known as "Miss Showbusiness." In 1939, she absolutely captivated audiences when, although just seventeen years old, she delivered a masterful performance in *The Wizard of Oz*. She followed it up with a recurring role as sweet Betsey Booth in the Andy Hardy movies with Mickey Rooney. By the time the war ended, she was the world's favorite musical performer, having proven herself with well-received grown-up roles in popular films like *Girl Crazy* and *Meet Me in St. Louis*.

Garland wasn't what most people would describe as beautiful and, at just under five feet, had a hard time keeping excess weight off. While there is some difference of opinion as to who actually introduced Garland to amphetamines as a weight-loss method and when it happened, it's a matter of history that she quickly became hooked. Garland was conscious of her plain looks among the beautiful actresses on the MGM lot and did everything she could to compensate. The pressure was intense. Considered by many to be intensely emotional and prone to mood swings even before she started taking drugs, Garland became notoriously unreliable and unpredictable afterwards.

Shortly after the war, Garland married MGM director Vincente Minelli and gave birth to her first child, Liza. Following a short maternity leave (during which she is said to have been obsessed with losing the pounds pregnancy had left on her), Garland signed a contract with MGM for a then-unheard-of $300,000. The combined stress of being a wife, mother, television and movie star began to wear on her. She increased her dosage of amphetamines and, when they caused insomnia, started taking equally harsh barbiturates to get to sleep. Despite ever-mounting reports of strange and erratic behavior, she kept to her non-stop work schedule. Until March 1947, when she backed out of a deal to sing "On the Atchison, Topeka and the Santa Fe," one of her big hits, at the Academy Awards presentation. While shooting a musical number called "Voodoo" for her new film *The Pirate* in April 1947, Garland suddenly stopped singing and started screaming "They're going to kill me!" over and over again. She collapsed into a heap of tears, punching and kicking at those who came to her aid. Security officers attempted to lead her away, but she broke free and ran headlong into a group of milling extras, screaming and begging for Benzedrine. She was back at work within a month, but repeatedly required time off throughout the filming.

The Pirate would become the only film she ever did for MGM that did not turn a profit.

After that, things got much worse for Garland. She was fired from *The Barkleys of Broadway* in 1949 because of missed rehearsals and was replaced by Ginger Rogers. A year later, after completing just two musical numbers in *Annie Get Your Gun*, she missed a series of rehearsals again and was replaced by Betty Hutton. MGM was out of patience. But Garland was a proven commodity and still had the ability to draw huge legions of fans. She got another chance later that year when she filmed *Summer Stock* with MGM's B-unit—a collection of less accomplished writers, directors and technicians. Normally, it would be considered a huge insult to a star of her caliber, but Garland had a great desire to get back to the top. And she staked a powerful claim. Although not all of her fans agree, many consider her number "Get Happy" with co-star Gene Kelly the best work of her entire career. Convinced she was back on track, the producers gave her the lead role in *Royal Wedding* after a pregnancy forced June Allyson to drop out, but was suspended by the studio when she started blowing off rehearsals again. Two days later, she cut her throat with a piece of broken glass.

It would be the first of many suicide attempts for Garland. Over the years, she would make many comebacks and suffer many personal tragedies, including four failed marriages. Despite never becoming unpopular, selling tons of records, hundreds of television appearances and even hosting her own critically acclaimed variety series on CBS, Garland could never escape her drug problems. In her final years, she was virtually homeless, staying at friends' houses and even sometimes sleeping outside. After she was fired from the 1967 film *Valley of the Dolls*, she rarely worked. Her fifth husband—Mickey Deans, a nightclub manager who met her while delivering drugs—found her body on in the bathroom of their London apartment on June 29, 1969. Coroner Dr. Robert Pocock determined that the forty-seven-year-old Garland died of a severe barbiturate overdose.

While amphetamines were popular with celebrities a few generations back, almost nobody famous has even admitted to meth use—although many, like guitarist Eddie Van Halen, have been accused of it when they have taken on an unhealthy appearance. The most notable admitted celebrity meth user thus far has been Jodie Sweetin. If you haven't heard of her, she's most famous for having played Stephanie Tanner on the long-running, if critically reviled, television series *Full House*. After the show wrapped in 1995, Sweetin (perhaps too strongly associated with the series) had a hard time finding work. Unemployed and bored, Sweetin turned to drugs in her late teens, eventually becoming a meth addict about the time she turned twenty. Despite being married to a police officer, who she said was unaware of her drug use, she started taking meth as part of her daily routine. According to her publicist, her former *Full House* castmates staged an intervention and convinced her to enter rehab.

Months later, Sweetin, now divorced, clean, and twenty-four years old and desperately eager to get her career back on track, in September 2005 signed on to host Fuse TV's *Pants-Off Dance Off*, a game show in which contestants must strip to win prizes.

TV Guide called it "the dumbest show in television history."

Waking up every morning knowing you're the host of *Pants-Off Dance Off* may seem like punishment overkill, but Sweetin should nevertheless be commended for admitting to and over-coming her addiction and having the courage to rejoin the work world, in whatever capacity. The fact that she is alone among celebrities (at least outside of the porn world) who have admit-ted to meth abuse, however, let alone beaten it, is an indicator of how little public acceptance the drug has achieved, despite sur-veys and expert estimates that indicate millions use the drug.

"The simple fact is that meth is a different sort of drug than alcohol or pot," said Dianne, an emergency room nurse who regularly sees the affects of many different kinds of drugs. "I've never met anyone who was ever happy about taking meth."

Meth is following much the same pattern crack did. Hybrids derived from other moderately popular, but far less powerful stim-ulants, both meth and crack are cheap, highly addictive and pose considerable health risks. Both became very popular in a short period of time and were largely distributed by organized crime.

Crack started small, emerging in 1982 with the club scene in Miami, and received very little attention from authorities, who were at the time very much concerned with traditional pow-dered cocaine. As New York Senator Chuck Schumer, a Democrat, said in 2003 when he was researching the effects of meth and came up with the inevitable comparison: "Twenty years ago, crack was headed east across the United States like a

Mack truck out of control, and it slammed New York hard because we just didn't see the warning signs." Even if they had, there's probably very little they could have done. By 1986, crack was the dominant illegal drug in inner-city New York and could also be found in great amounts in twenty-eight states and the District of Columbia. The effect on culture was immediate. Crime rates leapt—in particular murder rates, as dealers would decide the boundaries of their retailing territory by shooting it out—and many people fled the cities for what they considered crack-free suburbs.

But that all changed in the middle nineties. Different people cite different reasons as to why crack flamed out in places like New York City—a cop I know said that "pretty well everyone who used it is either dead or in jail"—but nobody denies that it has. There is still crack use in the city, but it's far rarer than it was a few years ago. A pretty good indicator of crack's rise and fall in New York City can be seen in the number of murders committed there. In 1985, just as crack arrived, there were 1134 murders in the five boroughs. In 1990, the peak of the crack epidemic, there were 2245, despite a drop in overall population. That number fell to 633 in 1998, after crack use had been drastically reduced and fell to just 530 in 2005, even though the population of the city had risen significantly.

Crack is still popular in some other U.S. cities, like Buffalo, Atlanta, Detroit and Gary, Indiana, and those cities reflect that trend in high crime rates. Interestingly, Canadian cities, where crack use arrived much later, have not shown the decline large U.S. cities like New York, Miami, Chicago and Los Angeles have and some have shown an increase. Overall, however, crack use is a small fraction of what it was just a few years ago.

Contemporary meth use very clearly mirrors the spread of crack, although with different segments of the population. Both law enforcement and health care professionals tell me that the

IT DOESN'T MAKE YOU SMARTER

Reports of meth users engaging in dangerous and otherwise self-destructive behavior abound in the media.

- In July 2004, a 39 year-old man in LaFayette, Georgia, was talking to a social services worker who led him to his car to sign some forms and, as the social worker put it: "While he was sitting in the back seat, the front of his pants exploded." Investigators determined that the man — who had a meth lab inside his house—had hastily stuffed some red phosphorous and iodine in his pocket when he saw the government-issued car pull up. The resulting blast inflicted second- and third-degree burns on the man's legs and testicles.

- When a Missouri Highway Patrol officer pulled over a 1990 Ford Thunderbird in July 2006 for a routine traffic stop, he was surprised to see the car's occupants flee on foot. A routine search of the car revealed $12,000 in cash and a homemade but fully functional four-foot-long rocket stuffed with more than two pounds on meth. The suspects, who were soon chased down and arrested, activated the missile, but forgot to connect it to the battery.

- In Decatur, Tennessee, the owner of an adult novelty store recognized a couple who walked into his shop in May 2006. It took a while for him to make the connection, but when he remembered that he had seen them on a surveillance video while they were burglarizing his store, he phoned the police. When they were arrested, police found a digital scale, Vicodin pills, a well-used meth pipe and the couple's 3 year-old daughter in the back seat of their car.

- After a series of rooms in a Fort Bragg, California, motel were burglarized, investigators were surprised to find a note. It read: There was no one here to attend us guest in rm427. You even left the office unattended. You could have been burglarized. Your lucky I didn't steele." Oddly, it was signed with the writer's full name. When police tracked him and his girlfriend down, they arrested the couple for burglary and possession of meth.

- A man showed up at a Portland, Oregon, hospital emergency room in September 2002 complaining of severe headaches. When doctors looked at his X-rays, they were shocked to see no fewer than 12 nails in his head. When they confronted him after a long and painstaking surgery, he tried to escape and then told them that he'd had an accident with a nail gun. After a series of interviews, he finally revealed that he was coming down from a meth high and was trying to kill himself with his nail gun.

Sources: Akron Beacon-Journal, Macon Telegraph, Columbia Daily Tribune, Decatur Daily, Associated Press and The Seattle Times.

overwhelming majority of meth users come from what they consider targeted populations. In the places it began, like small-town California, Arizona and British Columbia, meth use has saturated the market of potential users, much as crack did in New York. But the fact is that meth use is still spreading, at least geographically.

In recent years, meth has invaded places where it had been virtually unknown. "It started with our middle- and upper-class youth," said detective sergeant Jerome Engele, of the integrated crime unit in Saskatoon, where the drug started appearing in 2001. "But now it's used by people from all walks of life." The drug is still traveling eastward and northward and is expanding in Ontario and much of eastern North America.

Many people have told me that they fear meth will continue to expand and entrench itself into our culture. They fear that it could become more commonplace and accepted, like marijuana, and inch its way towards legality.

That's almost certainly not going to happen. People are just too smart for that.

Most people, anyway.

BRIAN AND I leave the donut shop just after I notice that the young man by the door has left with one of the other customers. As we are walking down a deserted residential street and turn into the parking garage where I left my car, Brian pulls out his bullet. Ever since I met him, he's been arguing that, without trying meth, I don't really have the credibility to write about it. And he's not the only one. Lots of people who I've discussed this project with have encouraged me to try meth, to give myself a better perspective.

And I do fit some of the aspects of the target audience. I don't have the energy and motivation that I used to and really could stand to lose a few pounds. I'm tempted, but only for a moment. I've just seen too much and know too much. When I look at Brian, I realize that there are negatives in my life, but I am way better off than him. Far better off I'd say than any meth user I've ever met. My life might not be perfect, but it's certainly not fucked up beyond redemption, like so many meth users I've seen.

The scare tactics have worked. I'm not going to try meth and it has nothing to with anything any cop, politician, advocate or physician has told me or shown me. I'm not going to try meth because I've seen up close what it does, not just in isolated cases, but consistently.

Brian is disappointed.

WHEN I VISIT ERIN again, she's back at work. Not at the same place she was working when I met her, though. Too many bad memories, she said. Instead, she is working at a car parts store. It pays more and it's closer to home. One of the guys who works there is an old friend of Justin's, but he doesn't seem to her like he uses meth.

"There's no way Donnie's on meth." She lowers her voice to a whisper. "He's fat."

When I ask her about Justin, she's appears, for the first time since I've met her, a picture of parental pride. "He's out of rehab and doing very well." She practically beams as she says it. When I talk to her about her son, she spits out all the well-known maxims of the rehab industry—"one day at a time" and how "you're never really cured, just in recovery." Justin has a job at the very flea market where he used to hock Erin's stolen possessions. She became such a regular that she got to know the manager and convinced him to give her son a job. He doesn't do much, just clean up and move stuff around, but she says it's a start. The manager pays his salary directly to Erin and his job is conditional on him staying off drugs.

As a boy, Justin wanted to be a veterinarian. He was a pretty decent guitar player as a teenager and used to write poetry that he didn't know his mother read. Today he is a functional illiterate who spends his days scrubbing toilets and picking up heavy things for minimum wage.

"Things could be worse, a lot worse," says Erin. "At least he's not stealing and he's not violent—it's like the bad part of his brain has been removed."

It's an incomplete simile. There's a lot more than just the "bad part" gone. Justin really doesn't do much of anything anymore. He works, he sleeps, he eats—all at the urging of his mother because he never really knows when he has to do these things. He's been cut out of the decision-making process of his own life.

Recently, Erin says, she found him staring off into space. She asked him what he was doing.

He told her.

"Dreaming of drugs."

Amped Bached Bob Buzzed Cranked up Foiled Fried Gacked Gassed Geeked Gurped Heated In psychosis Jacked Lit Pissed Pumped Ripped Rollin' Scattered Sparked Speeding Spin-Jo Spracked Spun or monkey spun Stoked Twacked Tweeked Twisted Wide awake or wide open Wired Worked Zipped Basehead Battery bender Cluckers or chicken-headed clucks Crackhead Crankster or cranker Doorknobber Fiend Geek or geeker Go-go loser Jibby jibby bear or jibbhead Loker Neck creature Shadow people Sketcher sketch cookie sketch monster or sketchpad Spin doctor or spinster Tweakers Wiggers Amped Bached Bob Buzzed Cranked up Foiled Fried Gacked Gassed Geeked Gurped Heated In psychosis Jacked Lit Pissed Pumped Ripped Rollin' Scattered Sparked Speeding Spin-Jo Spracked Spun or monkey spun Stoked Twacked Tweeked Twisted Wide awake or wide open Wired Worked Zipped Basehead Battery bender Cluckers or chicken-headed clucks Crackhead Crankster or cranker Doorknobber Fiend Geek or geeker Go-go loser Jibby jibby bear or jibbhead Loker Neck creature Shadow people Sketcher sketch cookie sketch monster or sketchpad Spin doctor or spinster Tweakers Wiggers Amped Bached Bob Buzzed Cranked up Foiled Fried Gacked Gassed Geeked Gurped Heated In psychosis Jacked Lit Pissed Pumped Ripped Rollin' Scattered Sparked Speeding Spin-Jo Spracked Spun or monkey spun Stoked Twacked Tweeked Twisted Wide awake or wide open Wired Worked Zipped Basehead Battery bender Cluckers or chicken-headed clucks Crackhead Crankster or cranker Doorknobber Fiend Geek or geeker Go-go loser Jibby jibby bear or jibbhead Loker Neck creature Shadow people Sketcher sketch cookie sketch monster or sketchpad Spin doctor or spinster Tweakers Wiggers Amped Bached Bob Buzzed Cranked up Foiled Fried Gacked Gassed Geeked Gurped Heated In psychosis Jacked Lit Pissed Pumped Ripped Rollin' Scattered Sparked Speeding Spin-Jo Spracked Spun or monkey spun Stoked Twacked Tweeked Twisted Wide awake or wide open Wired Worked Zipped Basehead Battery bender Cluckers or chicken-headed clucks Crackhead Crankster or cranker Doorknobber Fiend Geek or geeker Go-go loser Jibby jibby